Communications
in Computer and Information Science   137

Luo Qi (Ed.)

Parallel and Distributed Computing and Networks

International Conference, PDCN 2010
Chongqing, China, December 13-14, 2010
Revised Selected Papers

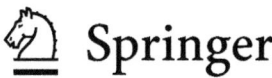 Springer

Volume Editor

Luo Qi
Wuhan Institute of Technology
Wuhan, Hubei, China
E-mail: witluo@ieee.org

ISSN 1865-0929   e-ISSN 1865-0937
ISBN 978-3-642-22705-9   ISBN 978-3-642-22706-6 (eBook)
DOI 10.1007/978-3-642-22706-6
Springer Heidelberg Dordrecht London New York

Library of Congress Control Number: 2011932349

CR Subject Classification (1998): C.2.1, C.2, D.2, C.1.4, C.2.4, D.4.7

Typesetting: Camera-ready by author, data conversion by Scientific Publishing Services, Chennai, India

Printed on acid-free paper

Springer is part of Springer Science+Business Media (www.springer.com)

Preface

We are delighted to present the proceedings of the 2010 International Conference on Parallel and Distributed Computing and Networks (PDCN 2010) held in Chongqing, China, during 13–14 December, 2010. The objective of PDCN is to provide a forum for researchers, educators, engineers, and government officials involved in the general areas of parallel and distributed computing and networks to disseminate their latest research results and exchange views on the future research directions of these fields.

This year, PDCN 2010 invited high-quality recent research results in the areas of parallel and distributed computing and networks. The conference provided an opportunity for academic and industry professionals to discuss the latest issues and progress in the area. Furthermore, we expect that the conference and its publications will be a trigger for further related research and technology improvements in this important subject.

PDCN 2010 included presentations of contributed papers and state-of-the-art lectures by invited keynote speakers. The conference brought together leading researchers, engineers and scientists from around the world. We would like to thank the Program Chairs, organization staff, and the members of the Program Committees for their hard work. Special thanks go to Springer.

We belive that PDCN 2010 was successful and enjoyable. We look forward to seeing all of you next year at PDCN 2011.

Qi Luo

Organization

Honorary Conference Chairs

Chin-Chen Chang   IEEE Fellow, Feng Chia University, Taiwan
Jun Wang   The Chinese University of Hong Kong, Hong Kong
Chris Price   Aberystwyth University, UK

Organizing Chairs

Honghua Tan   Wuhan Instititue of Technology, China
Junqiao Xiong   Wuhan University, China
Fan Yang   Wuhan Institute of Technology, China
Zhifang Yang   Wuhan Institute of Technology, China

Program Chairs

Wang Bin   Northeastern University, China
Qi Luo   Wuhan Instititue of Technology, China

Publication Chair

Qi Luo   Wuhan Instititue of Technology, China

International Program Committee

Ying Zhang   Wuhan Uniersity, China
Xueming Zhang   Beijing Normal University, China
Peide Liu   Shangdong Economic University, China
Dariusz Krol   Wroclaw University of Technology, Poland
Jason J. Jung   Yeungnam University, Republic of Korea
Paul Davidsson   Blekinge Institute of Technology, Sweden
Cao Longbing   University of Technology Sydney, Australia
Huaifeng Zhang   University of Technology Sydney, Australia
Qian Yin   Beijing Normal University, China

Reviewers

Dehuai Zeng   Shenzhen University, China
Qihai Zhou   Southwestern University of Finance and Economics,
                             China
Yongjun Chen   Guangdong University of Business Studies, China

Luo Qi	Wuhan Institute of Technology, China
Zhihua Zhang	Wuhan Institute of Physical Education, China
Yong Ma	Wuhan Institute of Physical Education, China
Zhenghong Wu	East China Normal University, China
Chen Jing	Wuhan University of Technology, China
Xiang Kui	Wuhan University of Technology, China
Li Zhijun	Wuhan University of Technology, China
Zhang Suwen	Wuhan University of Technology, China
Shufang Li	Beijing University, China
Tianshu Zhou	George Mason University, USA
Bing Wu	Loughborough University, UK
Huawen Wang	Wuhan University, China
Zhihai Wang	Beijing Jiaotong University, China
Ronghuai Huang	Beijing Normal University, China
Xiaogong Yin	Wuhan University, China
Jiaqing Wu	Guangdong University of Business Studies, China
Xiaochun Cheng	Middlesex University, UK
Jia Luo	Wuhan University of Science and Technology Zhongnan Branch, China
Toshio Okamoto	University of Electro-Communications, Japan
Kurt Squire	University of Wisconsin-Madison, USA
Xianzhi Tian	Wuhan University of Science and Technology Zhongnan Branch, China
Alfredo Tirado-Ramos	University of Amsterdam, The Netherlands
Bing Wu	Loughborough University, UK
Yanwen Wu	Central China Normal University, China
Harrison Hao Yang	State University of New York at Oswego, USA
Dehuai Zeng	Shenzhen University, China
Weitao Zheng	Wuhan University of Technology, China
Qihai Zhou	Southwestern University of Finance and Economics, China
Tianshu Zhou	George Mason University, USA
Shao Xi	Nanjing University of Posts and Telecommunication, China
Xueming Zhang	Beijing Normal University, China
Peide Liu	Shandong Economic University, China
Qian Yin	Beijing Normal University, China
Zhigang Chen	Central South University, China
Hoi-Jun Yoo	Korea Advanced Institute of Science and Technology, Korea
Chin-Chen Chang	Feng Chia University, Taiwan
Jun Wang	The Chinese University of Hong Kong, Hong Kong

Table of Contents

A Robust Zero-Watermark Algorithm Based on Singular Value Decomposition and Discreet Cosine Transform

Tianyu Ye

College of Information & Electronic Engineering, Zhejiang Gongshang University,
Hangzhou 310018, P.R. China
flystu008@yahoo.com.cn

Abstract. A robust zero-watermark algorithm is proposed, which is based on singular value decomposition and discreet cosine transform. The image is firstly spilt into non-overlapping blocks. Afterwards, every block is conducted with singular value decomposition, and its singular value matrix is transformed with discreet cosine transform. The robust zero-watermark sequence is derived from comparing the numerical relationship between two direct coefficients from adjacent blocks. Experimental results of robustness tests show that it has good robustness against various attacks.

Keywords: Digital watermarking, zero-watermark, singular value decomposition, discreet cosine transform, similarity.

1 Introduction

Intellectual property is of prime importance for authors, and the issue of intellectual property protection has gained great attentions from scholars. As we know, cryptography is a traditional way to protect the original works. Its drawback lies in that the original works turn out to be unreadable codes after encryption. How to achieve intellectual property protection and readability at the same time arises. Robust watermarking technology is naturally proposed to solve this problem. Robust watermarking technology can be realized in several domains, such as spatial domain, singular value decomposition (SVD), discreet cosine transform (DCT), discreet wavelet transform (DWT) and so on. Most robust watermark algorithms are realized in a single domain.

In order to solve the conflict between robustness and visual deterioration, the robust zero-watermark technology is firstly proposed by Wen Quan etc[1]. It essentially embed nothing into the original work, thus has perfect visual effect.

In this paper, it tries to design a robust zero-watermark algorithm in dual domains containing SVD and DCT. Experimental results of robustness tests show that it has good robustness against various attacks.

2 Mathematical Knowledge

SVD is a two-dimensional transform for a matrix. It is defined as follows:

L. Qi (Ed.): PDCN 2010, CCIS 137, pp. 1–8, 2011.
© Springer-Verlag Berlin Heidelberg 2011

$$\mathbf{H} = \mathbf{U}\mathbf{S}\mathbf{V}^{\mathrm{T}} \tag{1}$$

$$\mathbf{S} = \begin{bmatrix} \boldsymbol{\Sigma} & \mathbf{0} \\ \mathbf{0} & \mathbf{0} \end{bmatrix} \tag{2}$$

$$\boldsymbol{\Sigma} = diag(\lambda_1, \lambda_2, \lambda_3, \cdots, \lambda_r) \tag{3}$$

where $\mathbf{H}$ is the original $M \times N$ matrix, $\mathbf{U}$ is the left orthogonal matrix, $\mathbf{S}$ is the singular value matrix, $\mathbf{V}$ is the right orthogonal matrix, $\lambda_1, \lambda_2, \cdots, \lambda_r$ is its positive singular values, and r is its rank.

DCT is frequently used in image compression. Two-dimensional DCT is defined as follows:

$$C_{pq} = a_p a_q \sum_{m=0}^{M-1} \sum_{n=0}^{N-1} \mathbf{H}_{mn} \cos \frac{\pi(2m+1)p}{2M} \cos \frac{\pi(2n+1)q}{2N} \tag{4}$$

$$a_p = \begin{cases} \dfrac{1}{\sqrt{M}}, & p = 0 \\ \sqrt{\dfrac{2}{M}}, & 1 \le p \le M-1 \end{cases} \tag{5}$$

$$a_q = \begin{cases} \dfrac{1}{\sqrt{N}}, & q = 0 \\ \sqrt{\dfrac{2}{N}}, & 1 \le q \le N-1 \end{cases} \tag{6}$$

where C_{pq} is the DCT coefficient, $0 \le p \le M-1$ and $0 \le q \le N-1$.

3   The Production of Original Robust Zero-Watermark Sequence from the Original Image

The size of original image $\mathbf{H}$ is $N \times N$. The original roust zero-watermark sequence $\mathbf{W}$ is derived from it according to the following steps:

A1: First, split $\mathbf{H}$ into non-overlapping blocks of size $m \times m$. Every block is denoted as $\mathbf{H}_k$.

A2: Second, perform SVD on $\mathbf{H}_k$, and the singular value matrix of $\mathbf{H}_k$ is denoted as $\mathbf{S}_k$.

A3: Afterwards, transform $\mathbf{S}_k$ with DCT, and the direct coefficient (DC) of $\mathbf{S}_k$ is denoted as D_k.

A4: Finally, derive the original robust zero-watermark sequence $\mathbf{W}$ from comparing the numerical relationship between two DC coefficients from adjacent blocks, i.e.,

$$\text{If} \quad D_{2i-1} \geq D_{2i}$$

$$\mathbf{W}_i = 0;$$

else

$$\mathbf{W}_i = 1 \tag{7}$$

where $\mathbf{W}_i$ is the ith bit of $\mathbf{W}$, and $i = 1, 2, \cdots, \dfrac{N^2}{2m^2}$.

4 The Extraction of Robust Zero-Watermark Sequence from the Attacked Image

It derives the roust zero-watermark sequence from the attacked image $\mathbf{H}^\Lambda$ according to the following steps:

A1: First, split $\mathbf{H}^\Lambda$ into non-overlapping blocks of size $m \times m$. Every block is denoted as $\mathbf{H}_k^\Lambda$.

A2: Second, perform SVD on $\mathbf{H}_k^\Lambda$, and the singular value matrix of $\mathbf{H}_k^\Lambda$ is denoted as $\mathbf{S}_k^\Lambda$.

A3: Third, transform $\mathbf{S}_k^\Lambda$ with DCT, and the DC coefficient of $\mathbf{S}_k^\Lambda$ is denoted as D_k^Λ.

A4: Afterwards, derive the robust zero-watermark sequence $\mathbf{W}^\Lambda$ from comparing the numerical relationship between two DC coefficients from adjacent blocks, i.e.,

$$\text{If} \quad D_{2i-1}^\Lambda \geq D_{2i}^\Lambda$$

$$\mathbf{W}_i^\Lambda = 0;$$

else

$$\mathbf{W}_i^\Lambda = 1 \tag{8}$$

where $\mathbf{W}_i^\Lambda$ is the ith bit of $\mathbf{W}^\Lambda$.

A5: Finally, evaluate its robustness towards various attacks by similarity. Similarity between $\mathbf{W}$ and $\mathbf{W}^\Lambda$ is defined as

$$\eta = 1 - \left(\sum_{i=1}^{\frac{N^2}{2m^2}} \mathbf{W}_i \oplus \mathbf{W}_i^\Lambda \right) / \left(\frac{N^2}{2m^2} \right) \tag{9}$$

If $\eta \geq \tau$, the image owner is regarded to be legal, where τ is the threshold.

5 Experimental Results

Take grayscale images such as Lena, Sailboat and Frog for test images. They are shown in Figure 1, 2 and 3, respectively. Their amplitude is 512×512. The size of block is 8×8, thus the length of zero-watermark sequence is 2048 bit. Various attacks are imposed to test its robustness in this section. PSNR, whose unit is dB, is used to evaluate the visibility discrepancy between **H** and $\mathbf{H}^{\Lambda}$. PSNR is placed below "/" and similarity is placed above "/" in each table.

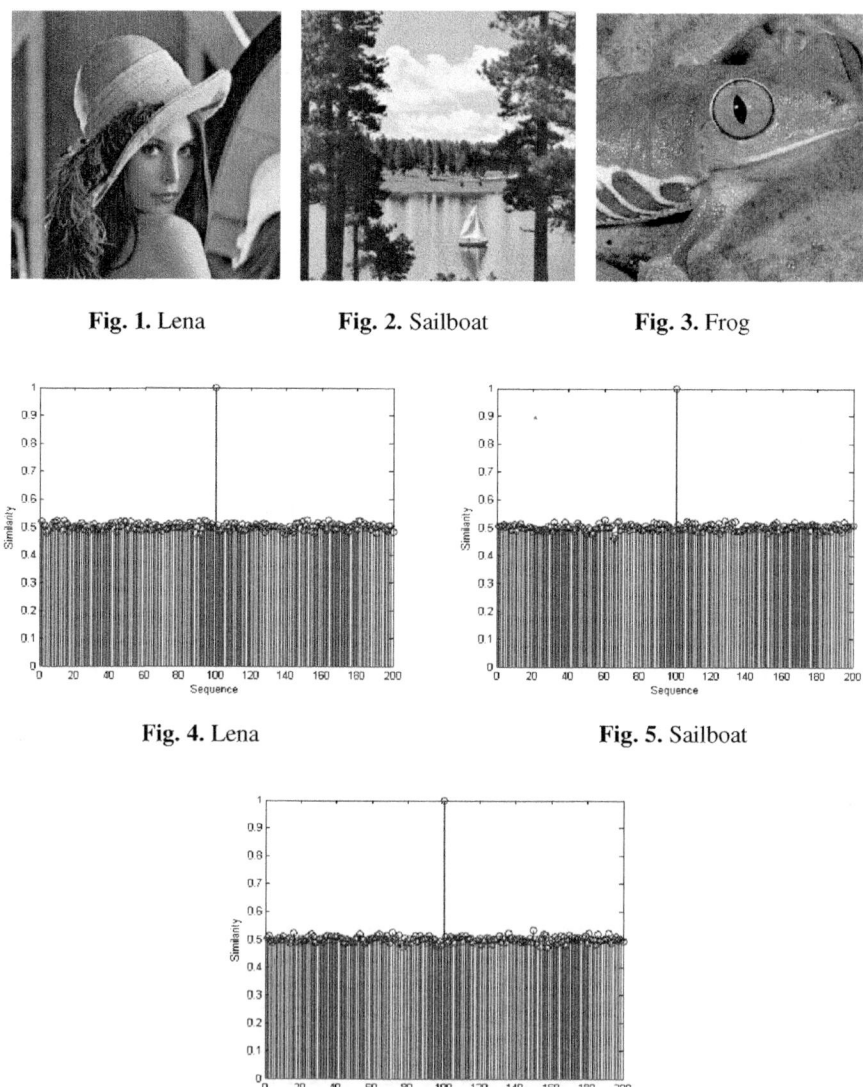

Fig. 1. Lena   **Fig. 2.** Sailboat   **Fig. 3.** Frog

Fig. 4. Lena   **Fig. 5.** Sailboat

Fig. 6. Frog

It produces 199 random uniform sequences and calculates their similarity to the original robust zero-watermark sequences from Lena, Sailboat and Frog. The results are shown in Figure 4, 5 and 6, respectively, where the 100th sequence is the original robust zero-watermark sequence. It is easy to find out that almost all results fluctuate around 0.5 in an extremely small range. Thus, it is enough to set the threshold equal to 0.75.

Various attacks are imposed to test its robustness in the following part.

(1) Gaussian noise
Gaussian noise is added to the original images, and the robustness test results are shown in Table 1.

Table 1. Gaussian noise

Image	Variance	
	0.001	0.003
Lena	0.9004 / 29.9743	0.8560 / 25.2360
Sailboat	0.8853 / 30.0083	0.8433 / 25.2920
Frog	0.8955 / 30.0148	0.8599 / 25.2896

(2) Salt&Pepper Noise
Salt&Pepper noise is added to the original images, and the robustness test results are shown in Table 2.

Table 2. Salt&Pepper noise

Image	Intensity	
	0.003	0.005
Lena	0.9268 / 30.8848	0.8818 / 28.6778
Sailboat	0.9282 / 30.0130	0.8950 / 27.7319
Frog	0.9058 / 31.0437	0.8584 / 28.6574

(3) Median Filter
Median filter is imposed to the original images, and the robustness test results are shown in Table 3.

Table 3. Median filter

Image	Window size	
	2×2	5×5
Lena	0.9531 / 29.2505	0.9453 / 30.9089
Sailboat	0.9185 / 26.6885	0.9082 / 26.3318
Frog	0.8755 / 24.8450	0.8140 / 23.6367

(4) Cropping
Cropping is imposed to the original images, and the robustness test results are shown in Table 4.

Table 4. Cropping

Image	Size	
	1/16 upper left corner	1/8 upper left corner
Lena	0.9561 / 17.2873	0.9131 / 14.7612
Sailboat	0.9683 / 14.3895	0.9429 / 13.4705
Frog	0.9712 / 17.8293	0.9390 / 14.7391

(5) JPEG Compression
JPEG compression is imposed to the original images, and the robustness test results are shown in Table 5.

Table 5. JPEG compression

Image	Quality factor				
	50	40	30	20	10
Lena	0.9463 / 35.4778	0.9399 / 34.8008	0.9316 / 33.9524	0.8950 / 32.6331	0.8306 / 30.0878
Sailboat	0.9233 / 31.9703	0.9126 / 31.4001	0.8960 / 30.6628	0.8691 / 29.5084	0.8315 / 27.2563
Frog	0.8535 / 27.7083	0.8589 / 27.2425	0.8530 / 26.7242	0.8516 / 25.9929	0.8081 / 24.6567

(6) Right Shifting
Right shifting means to right shifting the whole image several columns, filling the left blank columns with black and dropping the right columns. Right shifting is imposed to the original images, and the robustness test results are shown in Table 6.

Table 6. Right shifting

Image	Column number	
	1	2
Lena	0.9346 / 26.0819	0.8647 / 21.9928
Sailboat	0.9077 / 24.2405	0.8271 / 20.2930
Frog	0.8730 / 20.9542	0.7998 / 19.3739

(7) Random Column Removal
Random column removal refers to shifting left column-by-column from the first right column of the deleted column, and filling the right blank columns with black. Random column removal is imposed to the original images, and the robustness test results are shown in Table 7.

Table 7. Random column removal

Image	Column number	
	1	3
Lena	0.9644 / 27.8775	0.8911 / 21.8538
Sailboat	0.9404 / 26.4461	0.8555 / 20.7668
Frog	0.9199 / 23.1865	0.8359 / 20.4660

(8) Scaling
Scaling is imposed to the original images, and the robustness test results are shown in Table 8.

Table 8. Scaling

Image	Proportion	
	First lessen to 80%, then magnify to 125%	First lessen to 50%, then magnify to 200%
Lena	0.9390 / 25.7135	0.9365 / 27.9679
Sailboat	0.9082 / 23.6930	0.8970 / 24.1191
Frog	0.8477 / 21.7598	0.8174 / 22.5125

According to the above tests, it turns out that the suggested algorithm has good robustness against various attacks.

6 Conclusions

In this paper, a robust zero-watermark algorithm based on SVD and DCT is proposed. The image is firstly spilt into non-overlapping blocks. Afterwards, every block is conducted with SVD, and its singular value matrix is transformed with DCT. The robust zero-watermark sequence is derived from comparing the numerical relationship between two DC coefficients from adjacent blocks. It essentially embeds nothing into the original image, thus it has good visual effect. Experimental results of robustness tests show that it has good robustness against various attacks.

References

1. Wen, Q., Sun, Y.-f., Wang, S.-x.: Concept and Application of Zero-watermark. Acta Electronica Sinica 31(2), 214–216 (2003)
2. Liu, R.-z., Tan, T.-n.: SVD Based Digital Watermarking Method. Acta Electronica Sinica 29(2), 168–171 (2001)
3. Tsai, M.-j., Hung, H.-y.: DCT and DWT-based Image Watermarking by Using Subsampling. In: Proc. of the 24th International Conference on Distributed Computing Systems Workshops, MNSA (ICDCSW 2004), Hachioji, Tokyo, Japan, pp. 184–189 (2004)

4. Huang, D.-r., Liu, J.-f.: An Embedding Strategy and Algorithm for Image Watermarking in DWT Domain. Journal of Software 13(7), 1290–1297 (2002)
5. Lahouari, G., Ahmed, B., Mohammad, K.I., Said, B.: Digital Image Watermarking Using Balanced Multiwavelets. IEEE Trans. on Signal Processing 54(4), 1519–1536 (2006)
6. Sharkas, M., ElShafie, D., Hamdy, N.: A Dual Digital-image Watermarking Technique. In: Proc. of 3rd World Enformatika Conference (WEC 2005), Istanbul, Turkey, pp. 136–139 (2005)
7. Xu, L.-l., Wang, Y.-m.: Robust Digital Watermarking Scheme Resistant to Gaussian Noise, Geometric Distortion and JPEG Compression Attacks. Journal of Electronics & Information Technology 30(4), 933–936 (2008)
8. Niu, S.-z., Niu, X.-x., Yang, Y.-x., Hu, W.-q.: Data Hiding Algorithm for Halftone Images. Acta Electronica Sinica 32(7), 1180–1183 (2004)
9. Yuan, D.-y., Xiao, J., Wang, Y.: Study on the Robustness of Digital Image Watermarking Algorithms to Geometric Attacks. Journal of Electronics & Information Technology 30(5), 1251–1256 (2008)
10. Li, L.-d., Guo, B.-l., Biao, J.-f.: Spatial Domain Image Watermarking Scheme Robust to Geometric Attacks Based on Odd-even Quantization. Journal of Electronics & Information Technology 31(1), 134–138 (2009)

u-Traditional Market Model Based on 5W1H Context Aware Technology

Seoksoo Kim[*]

Department of Multimedia, Hannam University, Korea
sskim0123@naver.com

Abstract. A traditional market is losing its popularity while customers increasingly use online shops through the Internet or convenient large-scale discount stores and department stores. Although there have been some changes in facilities and PR events of a traditional market, its services are still not very convenient, failing to attract more customers. Therefore, this study suggests a u-traditional market mode to promote traditional markets. The system creates customized information and data through the context-aware(5W1H, Who, Where, What, When, Why, How) technology as well as heterogeneous sensors and RFID tags which collect real-time data of a traditional market and users' personal information.

Keywords: Context aware, Traditional market, 5W1H, USN.

1 Introduction

The governments of US, Japan, and Europe as well as corporations and major research institutes in those countries have recognized that the ubiquitous computer revolution is crucial to establishing their information and knowledge power, increasing competitiveness in the related industries.

Bill Gates, president of Microsoft(MS), the world's biggest software company, introduced 'SPOT(Smart Personal Object Technology)' as a new topic when he gave a keynote address at COMDEX. Here, a 'smart object' refers to a small electronic device such as an alarm clock, kitchen devices, stereo devices, and so on, which allow users to access online resources anytime and anywhere through Internet functions. That is, the term is another expression of ubiquitous, and one of the most important figures in the global IT industry announced the opening of the ubiquitous era. Likewise, ubiquitous has become a major issue in the world, and it is expected a new telecommunication environment will be established. For example, computers would become omnipresent but they are effectively integrated with users' environment so that their existence is not particularly noticed.

Meanwhile, a conventional market is losing its popularity while the number of large-scale discount stores and online shops keeps increasing. Although the government has introduced a special law for promoting the traditional market, customers avoid using the market due to its inconvenience [1].

---

[*] Corresponding author.

L. Qi (Ed.): PDCN 2010, CCIS 137, pp. 9–14, 2011.
© Springer-Verlag Berlin Heidelberg 2011

The term, "Context-aware" was first used by Schilit, Adamas, and Want. They described a context as an identity which differentiates a place, a human, and an object, or as a change in an environment including a human and an object [2]. Dey defined a context as a user's emotional state, attention, a location/direction, a date and time, and a human and an object in an environment to which a user belongs [3].

Therefore, this study suggests a u-traditional market model applying the RFID/ USN environment. The system creates customized information and data through the context-aware(5W1H, Who, Where, What, When, Why, How) technology with rules and cases that help to reason users' context as well as heterogeneous sensors which collect data of a traditional market and users' personal information or purchase patterns. Such data are used to offer accurate and realistic information through augmented reality functions of a smart phone. As a result, customers can compare prices of products available in a department store and a traditional market or come to know features and events provided only by a traditional market.

2 Augmented Reality and Handling Process

Augmented reality is a technology that enables view of a physical real-world that is augmented by virtual 3D generated imagery. It is a hybrid VR system where real-world is fused with virtual environment and researchers from US and Japan have taken a leading position in this technology since the latter part of 1990s. Traditionally, augmented reality has been widely used in areas such as remote medical diagnosis, broadcasting system, architectural design and manufacturing process management but recently, the technology has made headway into location-based service, mobile games and others. Augmented reality supplements physical real-world with virtual imagery information. For instance, using a smart phone as an example, when a phone's camera focuses on a particular building on a street, using GPS and geomagnetic sensors, it displays basic information on the building on the phone's screen.

We can expect to see someday when virtual animals and characters will greet and introduce certain areas to passerby. Although the basic premise of augmented reality is simple, its potential is limitless as all kinds of products and programs can be made to provide fun and interesting elements to users.

There are various types of augmented reality which includes a mark type where when a camera is fixated on a mark it provides 3D or 2D generated imagery on top of it. In contrast, there is also a non-mark type.

Recently, instead of augmented reality that uses non-mark, services where location-related information can be gathered by using GPS and geomagnetic sensors are gaining wide popularity[4].

3 Context-Awareness

A context-aware service aims to recognize the intention of users and his/her surrounding and provide a user-specific service. [5,6,7]

General context information can be largely divided into user context, physical environment context, computer system context, user-computer interaction history and other non-classified context. It can be further classified into users, IDs, physical body, space, time, and environment, where all elements from surrounding can be defined as context information. For information and services provided through context-awareness, it must have capability in deducing accurate information using collected context information[8].

Generally, context specifies information on 5W1H or Why, Where, What, When, Why, and How. If one closely reviews researches that use context, one sees that not all 5W1H elements are used, but rather, it is used in line with the objective of each application. Context involving Who/What that indicates resident/target respectively and location (Where) are.

It can be said that Who/What that indicates resident/target respectively and location (Where) are context that are widely used. In addition to Who, What, and Where, it uses "when did the event occur" (When) and "how did the event occur" (How). Additionally, using 5W1H, it recognizes "why did the event occur" (Why). As "Why" provides information on the reason why resident environment has changed, it can be said that it is a final context. When context is used at home, Who (resident aware), What (target aware), Where (resident and target's location), When (resident's entry time) and How & Why (resident's gesture and intention) are used. It can be said that based on this system, context-aware service is provided. To expand the range of services and realize context-aware service, the following matters must be considered first.

First, a network that enables uninterrupted sharing and transferring of information between devices should be constructed.

Second, hardware technology that can utilize this system should be secured.

Third, there should be hardware and software standardization for sharing and transferring of information between devices.

4 u-Traditional Market Promotion System Structure

First, the setting for hypothesized information on 5W1H(Who, Where, What, When, Why, How) is as follows.

Table 1. Hypothetic information on 5W1H (Who, Where, What, When, Why, How)

Who	Where	What	When	Why	How
Consumer	Resident and location of target	Awareness of target	Residents' entry time	Residents' gesture and intention	Generation method
Classification of consumers	Traditional market	Products of traditional market	Business hours of traditional market	Wanted products available? Is price reasonable?	General information and decision based on information of augmented reality

u-Traditional Market model structure is shown in figure 1 and handling process is as follows.

① Through sensor middleware, it gathers context information that can be collected from heterogeneous sensor and RFID tag from RFID/USN environment that are constructed in each store.

② Collected information is converted by a sensor middleware as required and saved into database.

③ Through the middleware, context-aware 5W1h elements and subsequent augmented reality is integrated and provides location-related information using GPS.

④ A web server, consisting of a smart phone and a context-aware service module, handles processes, and deduces data of context information saved in DB, and through web/mobile online markets and mobile devices where consumers can directly use, provides customized information and services.

⑤ Through mobile devices, consumers can use mobile and online market services ubiquitously and additionally, through a sensor network constructed in a traditional market, consumers can make the most of promotional events, location guide, and other dynamic services provided by sellers.

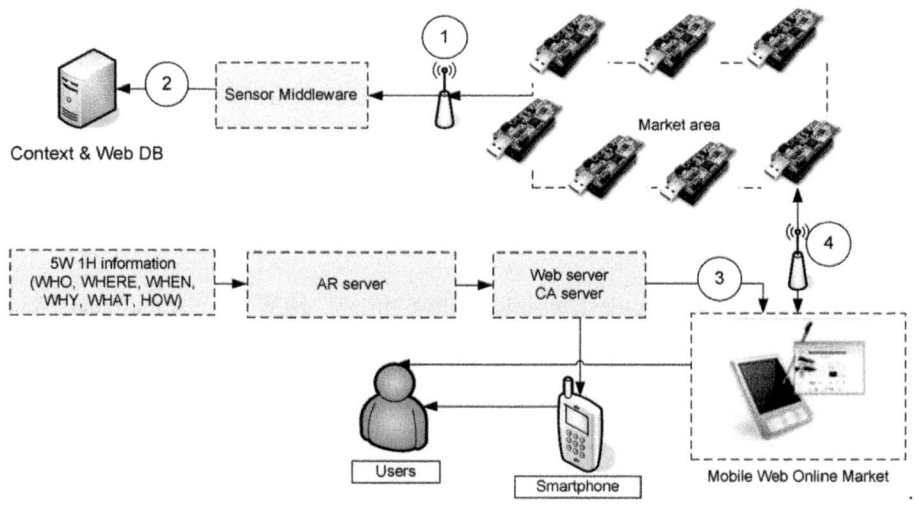

Fig. 1. u-CMIS model structure

As mentioned above in u-Traditional Market model, a web server, a key component that provides customized service to consumers, it processes and deduces data from DB. The handling process is shown in figure 2 and details are shown below[1].

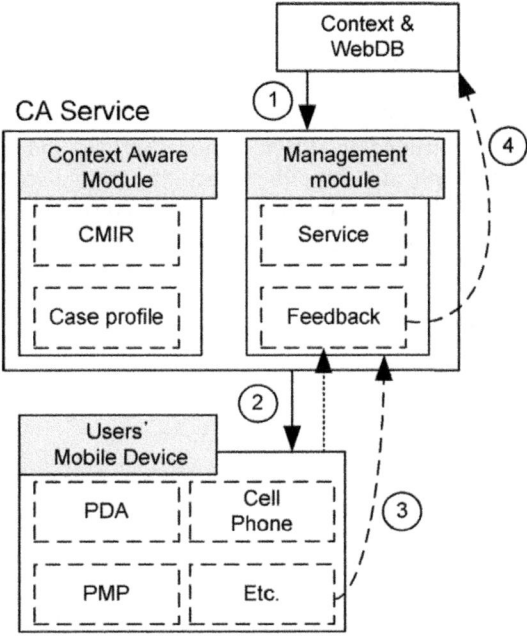

Fig. 2. Context deduction process

① Context-aware middleware, calls sensed data from DB and deduces Traditional Information Rule and profile information on consumers and traditional markets as required and generates customized information and services.

② Deduced customized information and services are provided to consumers through a management module.

③ Consumers can use a mobile phone to receive customized service and afterward, service feedback is sent to a module management.

④ The module management, in turn, manages the result of service feedback, and processes and saves confirmed data. Through this cycle, more data are added onto Traditional Information Rule and profile, enabling more accurate customized services.

5 Conclusion

With the advent of information age, a traditional market is losing its popularity while customers increasingly use online shops through the Internet or convenient large-scale discount stores and department stores. Although there have been some improvement in facilities and promotional events of a traditional market, its services are still not very convenient to customers, thus failing to attract more customers.

In light of above, u-Traditional Market model that this paper has proposed is a system where RFID/USN environment is applied within traditional markets. Using information on traditional markets collected by heterogeneous sensor, as well as consumer's personal information and spending patterns, it generates customized information and service in line with context-aware (5W1H: Who, Where, What, When, Why, How) technology.

The generated data using a smart phone can be used to provide real and accurate information via augmented reality, presenting products that have price advantage over department stores and introducing differentiated services and events of traditional market that cannot be duplicated by either convenient large-scale discount stores or department stores. In addition, through this model, consumers who frequent traditional markets will take a closer step to experiencing convenient ubiquitous city.

Acknowledgements

This paper has been supported by the 2010 Hannam University Research Fund.

References

1. Lim, J.-H., Kim, S.: Design of Context-Aware based u-CMIS System for Revitalization of Conventional Market, The Korea Academia-industrial cooperation, Autumn Conference (2009)
2. Schilit, B., Adams, N., Want, R.: Context-Aware Computing Applications. In: Proceedings of the Workshop on Mobile Computing System and Applications, pp. 85–90 (1994)
3. Chen, H., Finin, T., Joshi, A.: An Intelligent Broker for Context-Aware Systems. In: Adjunct Proceeding of Ubicomp 2003, pp. 12–15 (2003)
4. Lighthouse: AugmentedReality's Implementation Principle,
   http://blog.naver.com/lighthousede?Redirect=Log&logNo=70085196276
5. Sheng, Q.Z., Benatallah, B.: ContextUML: a UML-based Modeling language for model-driven development of context-aware Web services. In: Proceedings of the International Conference on Mobile Business, pp. 206–212 (2005)
6. Buchholz, T., Krause, M., Linnhoff-Popien, C., Schiffers, M.: CoCo: Dynamic Composition of Context Information. In: Proceedings of the First Annual International Conference on Mobile and Ubiquitous Systems: Networking and Services, pp. 335–343 (2004)
7. Chang, H., Lee, K.: Design of a Simulation-Based Development Tool for Context-Aware Service, Korea Society for Simulation, 2006 Autumn Conference, pp. 87–91 (2006)
8. Korea Electronics and Telecommunication Research Institute, RFID/USN Technolog trend (2008)
9. http://xenerdo.com/197

An HD Virtual Studio System Using Chroma Key

Seoksoo Kim[*]

Department of Multimedia, Hannam University, Korea
sskim0123@naver.com

Abstract. In this research, we used HDMI signals, designed for low-cost distribution, in order to implement an HD-definition virtual studio, processing analogue signals and broadcasting HD signals. In this way, one can carry out automatic extraction, play/record, and operation of a virtual camera, using chroma key In the system, moreover, users can deal with more conveniently loss of signals, color degradation, use of an HD output board, correction of a driver, and so on. Thus, the low-cost HD virtual studio system complies with the environmentally-friendly policies and helps users easily produce high-definition contents. As a result, use of an HD virtual studio becomes much easier while an online community can be promoted through a website sharing background contents, providing more high-quality contents and popularizing the related equipment.

Keywords: HD, Virtual studio, Chroma key, Synthesizing.

1 Introduction

Recently, more efforts have been made on research and application of U-learning, based on mobiles using wireless Internet. That is, the concept of 'ubiquitous' is being applied to education [1].

U-learning can bring the following changes. First, there will be a change in education places. In the ubiquitous era, individuals can receive education anywhere as remote education, a digital library, an outdoor classroom, and so on, are available and education places are not limited to geographically fixed places. So, various types of study resources will be easily available and accessed through mobile devices [2].

E-learning, which has been rapidly developed along with the increasing use of IT technology and the Internet since the late 1990's, began to grow at an outstanding rate in the 2000's and be considered the driving force for the IT market. Several years ago, the major figures of the IT industry, including John T. Chambers, chairman of CISCO which is a multinational IT corporation, already said that 'the next-generation killer application will be Internet-based education', emphasizing the importance of e-learning in the industry. Officers of Goldman Sachs and Anderson Consulting have also predicted that the higher value-added businesses in the 21C would be all based on e-learning.

So far, such e-learning industry has focused on educational contents produced by the one-sided demand of schools or companies. More recently, however, self-directed

---

[*] Corresponding author.

L. Qi (Ed.): PDCN 2010, CCIS 137, pp. 15–20, 2011.

learning, a new method of learning recently noted, allows learners to actively discuss a subject, increasing participation and maximizing learning effects. And cooperative learning, one of constructive learning methods, can be considered self-directed learning, for it encourages learners to discuss an issue and solve a problem together. Also, development of the wireless industry has increased the demand for learner-oriented educational services such as m-learning and u-learning. As a result, e-learning has been required to produce learner-oriented contents such as cooperative learning [3].

The size of the Korean e-learning market was 5.7 trillion won last year(2009) and the global market, 68,500 million dollars. And the CAGR(Compound Annual Growth Rate) of the global e-learning market was 22.4% in 2009.

The telecommunication infrastructure technology has achieved stabilization through the steady growth of the global e-learning market and its explosive growth in Europe and Asia. It's urgent that the government as well as the industry and schools come up with systematic responsive measures in view of the fact that large corporations have already begun to enter into and standardize the e-learning market.

According to Korea IDC, the size of the domestic SW/contents market is 23.4 trillion won in Korea while e-learning accounts for 2.5 trillion won of the market, increasing by 33% compared to the previous year. Although there has been a lot of efforts at developing HD equipment and a number of companies have actually released products, such device is very expensive and needs numerous additional devices (tracking/delay/Chromakey), making difficult its operation.

2 The Necessity of Research

Meanwhile, unlike broadcasting, cyber lectures using a virtual studio have not successfully applied various templates or screen technologies. It's maybe because a cyber studio is used in order to cut down expenses and less attention has been paid to effective screen composition. Most background templates applied to a virtual setting of a cyber lecture are space similar to a classroom in the real world or one with only minimum elements. In some cases, however, more complex 3D simulation technologies are used in order to create more various and realistic space for cyber lectures. That is, an increase in the quantity of cyber lectures has made production methods more various. In view of these trends, therefore, we have paid attention to cyber lectures using VR images [4].

2.1 Rising Demand for High-Resolution Contents Using a Virtual Studio System

Although HD digital conversion starts in 2012, a shift from SD definition to HD definition, most HD products are highly expensive and, thus, low-cost products shall be developed in order to replace HD virtual studio systems currently used by broadcasting companies. Though use of an HD virtual studio system requires expensive equipment such as an HD camera, the product suggested this study uses an HDMI output digital camera. Using an HDMI signal, designed for distribution, makes possible low-cost and high-definition HD images.

2.2 Significant Breakthrough in the E-Learning Industry Using Digital Contents of the Internet

E-learning introduces a new way of learning using virtual reality, not limited to the previous off-line methods using books or web-based contents, in order to encourage learners' interest and improve their concentration. The demand for this effective learning method is expected to keep rising.

2.3 Technical Aspects of a Virtual Studio System

Recently, 'Chroma key', a technique for showing images on the screen which actually do not exist in the studio', is frequently used.

The technique is commonly used for weather forecast broadcasts, films, virtual advertising, or English education programs for kids, as well as multi-media education system and monitoring systems. Chroma key requires highly expensive equipment and an HD virtual studio. In order to use the technique, a single-color background is used and a color range from one image is removed. Chroma key is sensitive to illumination and thus needs perfect illumination and background facility with high skills [5,6].

Chroma key is a technique for compositing two images(e.g. Image A and Image B) together and a color from Image B is made transparent, revealing Image A behind it. Since an object can be combined with the background, a learner feels the object is in the background, which may encourage his active participation. And such Chroma key technology is commonly used for professional systems [7].

An announcer stands in front of a background screen, which is a complementary color of a subject, and the images shot by a camera are later combined with weather maps or other information (Figure 1).

For compositing two images, a specific color(commonly, blue) is selected as a "key" and, in the principal image a pixel corresponding to the key is replaced by a pixel of another image. As depicted in Figure 1, the key is not a single color difference but a range of color differences.

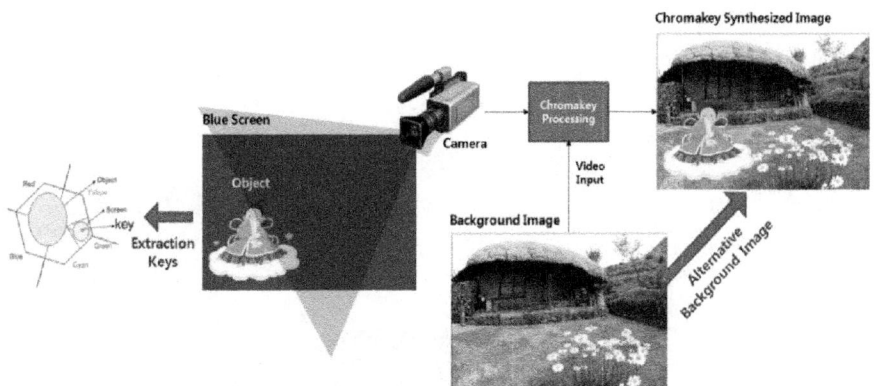

Fig. 1. Principle of Chromakey

3   Real-Time HD Virtual Studio Using Chroma Key

Recently, virtual studio has come to the fore as a new broadcasting method using the virtual reality technology. Although an man actually stands in a blue room, 3D images of a virtual background replace the setting. The virtual reality technology is used to simulate the virtual background in real time and produce an effect that the man exists in the virtual setting. Likewise, a virtual studio replaces a real setting and creates/operates a virtual setting. In order to make a high-quality composite screen, one must well design the FG image shooting setting and make the best use of the chroma-keying system. Particularly, in case of using a blue room that all walls and the floor are blue, one shall pay attention to preventing shades in the boundary surface. In the previous chroma-keying system, a camera shooting the FG image of an announcer should film in a fixed location. If a camera moves from side to side, the announcer would look like sliding from side to side in the fixed background. Also, if a camera moves forwards/backwards or zooms in/out, he would look larger or smaller. That is, a viewer can not feel that he speaks in front of maps or graphs but would feel that two separate men are in the screen. Therefore, if a camera moves, the location relation between FG and BG images is lost so that the camera must be fixed [8].

3.1   Real-Time HD Chromakey Logic Processing

Figure 2 shows how to extract chroma key while Figure 3 shows an example of a video process.

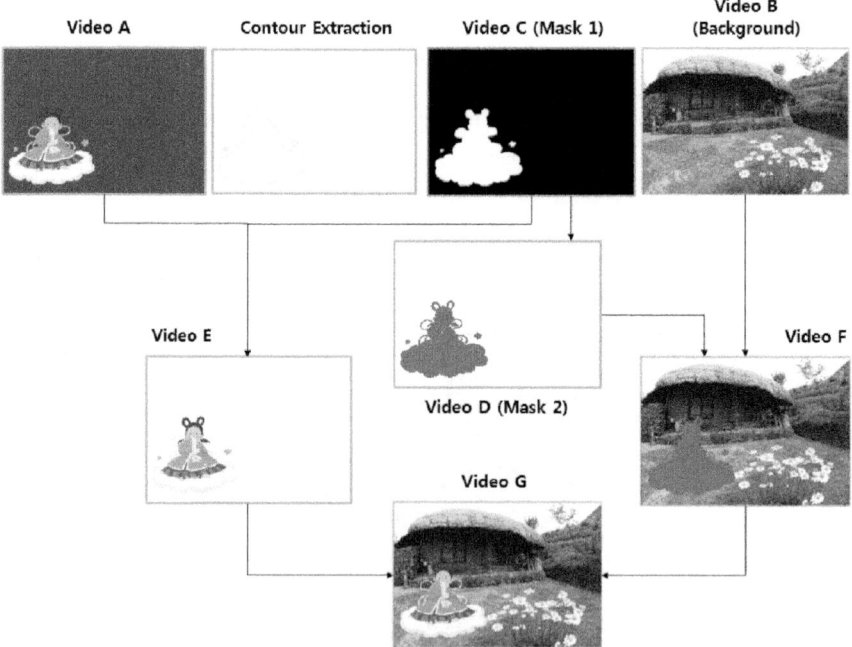

Fig. 2. Extraction of Chroma Key

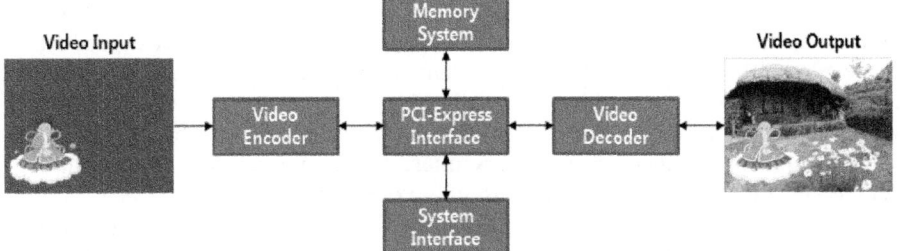

Fig. 3. Example of a Basic Video Process

- Use of a general-purpose board in order to solve a problem of a delayed period due to development of an HD video signal input board as well as development of an HD output board
- Use of SDK for chroma key of the input board
- Interface converting analogue and HDMI signals into digital
- Application of a capture board for extracting real-time chroma.

3.2 Development of a Real-Time 3D Background Rendering Program

Not only premiers but all video programs related with graphics including an editing program need a series of rendering processes. Each program has its own codec and, sometimes it should use another codec. Or an original file may change due to some effects. In this case, changed values shall be restored, which call for rendering.

- 3D background real-time rendering using a graphic card (nVIdia QuadroFX series)
- Offering of 2 shader stages for Geometry Tessellation
- Improved rendering quality and flexibility of Anti-Aliasing (per-sample fragment shader and programmable fragment shader input position)
- Data generation and drawing by external API such as OpenGL or OpenCL without interference of CPU.

3.3 Development of Hardware Driver Using Windows Driver Kit

- Development of a driver for Windows7, the latest version
- Windows Driver Foundation (WDF)
- Installable File System Kit (IFS Kit)
- Driver Test Manager (DTM)
- Later DTM was renamed to Windows Logo Kit (WLK) and separated from.

4 Conclusion

At present, cyber lectures using a virtual studio are not successful in utilizing various templates or screen processing techniques. Maybe, it's because a cyber studio is used in order to cut down expenses and less attention has been paid to effective screen composition. Most background templates applied to a virtual setting of a cyber lecture are space similar to a classroom in the real world or one with only minimum elements.

Although HD digital conversion starts in 2012, a shift from SD definition to HD definition, most HD products are highly expensive and, thus, low-cost products shall be developed in order to replace HD virtual studio systems currently used by broadcasting companies. Meanwhile, e-learning introduces a new way of learning using virtual reality, not limited to the previous off-line methods using books or web-based contents, in order to encourage learners' interest and improve their concentration. The demand for this effective learning method is expected to keep rising.

Recently, 'Chroma key', a technique for showing images on the screen which actually do not exist in the studio, is frequently used in various areas.

The technique is commonly used for weather forecast broadcasts, films, virtual advertising, or English education programs for kids, as well as multi-media education system and monitoring systems.

In this research, we used HDMI signals, designed for low-cost distribution, in order to implement an HD-definition virtual studio, processing analogue signals and broadcasting HD signals. In this way, one can carry out automatic extraction, play/record, and operation of a virtual camera, using chroma key. As a result, use of an HD virtual studio becomes much easier while an online community can be promoted through a website sharing background contents, providing high-quality contents and popularizing the related equipment.

Acknowledgements

This paper has been supported by the 2010 Hannam University Research Fund.

References

1. Kim, Y.: Suggestions for u-learning System based on the integrated education. Journal of the Korea Society of Korea Information 12(3) (2007)
2. Lee, J.-H., Choi, S.-K., Hwang, T., Cho, Y.-H.: P2P - Based Experience Learning Support System for U-Learning. Journal of The Korea Contents Association 5(6), 309–318 (2005)
3. Park, J., Kim, S.-H., Yang, J.: Empirical Studies on the Expression of Collective Intelligence and the Web2.0-based Collaborative e-Learning System. Journal of Korea Information Technology 8(8) (August 2010)
4. Bae, J.-A., Kim, Y.-J., Jeon, B.-H.: Cybercommunication academic society 25(3), 841–849 (2008)
5. Sang-Yeob, L., Heon-Sik, J.: A Study on the Implementation of Robust Automatic Adaptative Chroma-key Method. Journal of the Korea Society of Computer and Information 13(1), 21–27 (2008)
6. Kim, J.H., Choi II, D., Cho, W.Y.: A Study On The Implementation of Real Time Image Composition System Using Adaptive Algorithm. In: Conference on Information and Control Systems, vol. 25(2), pp. 569–572 (2003)
7. Kwak, S.-D., Chang, M.-S., Kang, S.-M.: Real time chromakey processing algorithms in general environment using the alpha channel. In: Korea Intelligent Information Systems Society 2010 Conference, vol. 20(1), pp. 188–189 (2010)
8. Ko, H.: Introduce of Virtual Studio. Korea Society Broadcast Engineers Magazine 2(2), 12–22 (1997)

A Secure Patient Information Access Scheme through Identity-Based Signcryption

Giovanni Cagalaban and Seoksoo Kim[*]

Department of Multimedia, Hannam University, 306-791 Daejeon, Korea
gcagalaban@yahoo.com, sskim0123@naver.com

Abstract. Privacy and security of patient health information has received worldwide attention as one of the critical research challenges due to its increasing access over the Internet in order to provide efficiency, accuracy, and availability of medical treatment. In this paper, we propose a novel efficient access scheme in order to provide various security characteristics for ubiquitous healthcare systems. In the ubiquitous environment, we deploy the recently developed concepts of identity-based signcryption in which the network effectively solves the problem of single point of failure in the traditional public-key infrastructure (PKI) supported system by providing key generation and key management services without any assumption of pre-fixed trust relationship between network devices.

Keywords: identity-based signcryption, access scheme, ubiquitous healthcare.

1   Introduction

The technological advancement of healthcare devices prompted existing healthcare information systems (HIS) to use networked computing systems for recording and accessing medical records [1]. Healthcare institutions are increasingly interested in sharing access of their information resources over the networked environment. However, transmission of sensitive patient medical information over the networked computer systems increases the risk of security and privacy.

Security considerations are needed in order to deal efficiently with the communication security issues described above. Much research has been done into creating key management schemes to meet the notion of security, authentication, and privacy. The security scheme is established on the basis of a secret group key that is shared among the privileged users, but is unknown to non-group members. However, the difficulty of managing cryptographic keys used for group communication arises from the dynamic membership change. Every time a member is added to or deleted from the group, the group controller must change the group key for backward or forward secrecy [2].

In this paper, we present a secure patient information access control scheme in a networked environment. In a ubiquitous healthcare environment, we deploy the recently developed concepts of identity-based signcryption in which the network effectively solves the problem of single point of failure in the traditional public-key infrastructure

---

[*] Corresponding author.

L. Qi (Ed.): PDCN 2010, CCIS 137, pp. 21–26, 2011.
© Springer-Verlag Berlin Heidelberg 2011

(PKI) supported system by providing key generation and key management services without any assumption of pre-fixed trust relationship between network devices. We implemented the proposed scheme by combining identity-based one-way encryption with message integrity or signature verification resolve the data or sender authentication problems.

2 Related Works

Related to healthcare information systems are the researches on dependability issues of ubiquitous computing in a healthcare environment which were analyzed by Bohn et. al. [3]. Security and privacy of RFID systems was introduced by Albrecht and McIntyre [4].

In order to shield transport and sharing of medical data and protect healthcare applications over the Internet there is a need of a suitable security scheme with appropriate structure, compatibility with PKI and PMI environments [6]. Blundo, et al. [7] propose several schemes that allow any group of parties to compute a common key, while being secure against collusion between some of them. For secure communication services, an identity-based authenticated broadcast encryption scheme was proposed by Mu et. al. [8]. Additionally, another identity-based ring signcryption scheme was proposed by Huang et. al. [9] based on cryptographic primitives for preserving privacy and authenticity. However, the concept was designed for a general ubiquitous computing and not directly applicable to addressing security issues in ubiquitous healthcare systems such as authentication, confidentiality, integrity and non-repudiation.

3 Identity-Based Signcryption Scheme

The concept of identity-based cryptography was proposed by Shamir [10] with the goal of simplifying certificate management in email system, thus avoiding the high cost of the public-key management and signature authentication in PKI supported cryptosystem. The basic idea is to find an approach wherein each entity's public key can be defined by an arbitrary string. In identity-based signcryption, a digital signature scheme is used for the authentication of messages and an encryption algorithm is used for the confidentiality of messages.

An identity-based signcryption scheme consists of the four algorithms: Setup, Extract, Signcrypt, and Unsigncrypt. Their functions are described below:

a. Setup: This algorithm generates the global public parameters *globalparams*, the master secret key s, and the master public key on the given security parameter k.

b. Extract: This algorithm generates a corresponding private secret key based on the given master secret key and the public key of the user.

c. Signcrypt: Assuming that A wishes to send a message m to B, this algorithm works by generating a ciphertext σ given the message m with its own secret key.

    d.   Unsigncrypt: Assuming that B receives a ciphertext σ from A, this algorithm is used to recover the message m from the ciphertext σ with its own secret key. This results in producing m, σ, and the identity of the sender A.

The concept of identity-based signcryption is applicable to patient information exchange where users may access sensitive patient information such as name, status of patient, and other identity which are used as their public key, thus there is no need to propagate this common information through the network. For ubiquitous healthcare systems, a private key generator (PKG), makes the master public key known to everyone which generates system parameters, and master public/private key pair. The master private key is only kept to itself.

The patient information access control scheme is aimed to provide a method for encrypting and signing data together in a way that is more efficient than using an encryption scheme combined with a signature scheme. Fig. 1 shows the flow of the access control scheme of the identity-based signcryption.

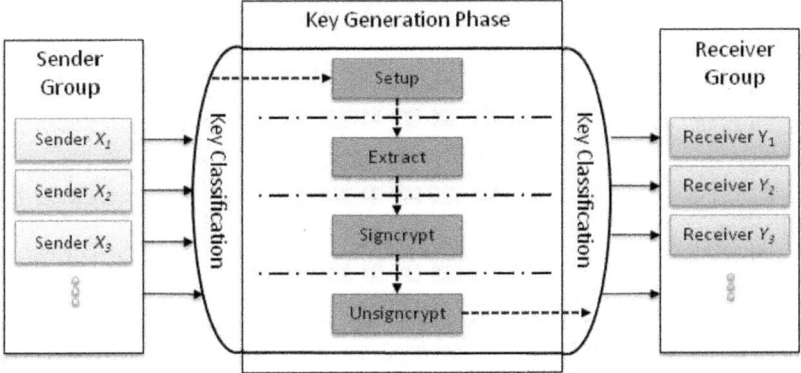

Fig. 1. Flow of Access Control Scheme

In a ubiquitous network environment, there are a centralized key server and multiple communication controllers for recording and accessing medical records of patients through networked computing systems as show in Fig. 2. A sender of a group is in charge of managing the group as a communication controller. The key server generates public parameters for the system and the keys for the network group senders and users.

The control access scheme in this paper does not rely on any assumption of underlying key management subsystem. There is no trusted authority to generate and distribute the public/private keys and there is no pre-built trust association between nodes in the network. All the keys used is generated and maintained in a self-organizing way within the network.

To describe the details of distributed key management and authentication mechanisms, first we assume the following parameters. We assume that $SS = \{\ \zeta_1,\ \zeta_2,...,\ \zeta_n\ \}$ represents the set of services in the network. Let $U = \{\ \psi_1,...,\ \psi_n\ \}$ be the universe of users. Let X_j denote the sender of $\zeta j \in SS$, and $Yj \subseteq U$ denote the set of members who can access the service ζj transmitted from Xj. For example, a member $\psi 1 \in Y1 \cap Y_2$ can access the broadcast services transmitted from X_1 and X_2 respectively. ID_U represents a public identity of U. For example, ID_{X_i} and ID_{Y_j} represent the identities of X_i and Y_j respectively.

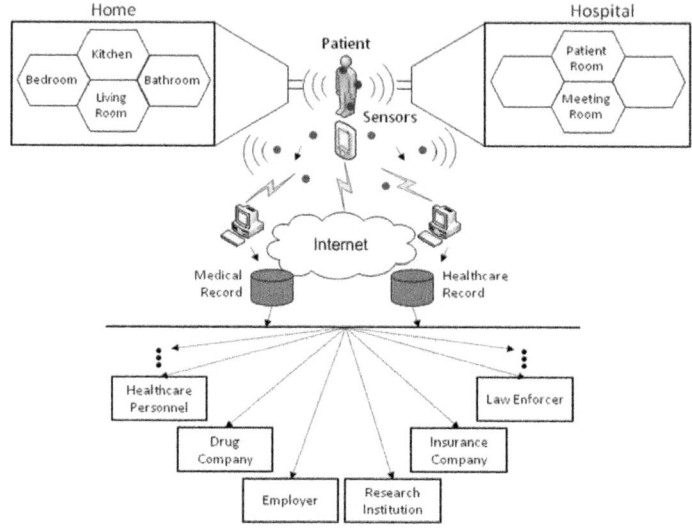

Fig. 2. Patient Information Access

Based on the assumptions made above, we can now construct the secure access control scheme for each of the algorithms of the identity-based signcryption. The cryptography in the proposed scheme makes use of a bilinear map $\gamma : \zeta_1 \times \zeta_1 \rightarrow \zeta_2$ where ζ_1, and ζ_2 are scalar services based on the order π.

For the Setup algorithm, the key server chooses a key generator PLK of ζ_1 and a random $s \in N*\pi$, and computes a master public key $PLKp \leftarrow sPLK$. The key server keeps s as a master secret key. Subsequently, the key server chooses cryptographic respective hash functions $H1 : \{0,1\}* \rightarrow \zeta 1$, $H2 : \{0,1\}* \rightarrow N*\pi$, $H3 : \zeta 2 \rightarrow \{0,1\}*$ and publishes parameters $globalparams = \{PLK, PLK_p, H_1, H_2, H_3\}$.

For the Extract algorithm, the key server extracts $T_{Xj} \leftarrow H_1 (ID_{Xj})$ and computes the private key $PVKXj \leftarrow sTXj$, $\forall Xj$ of $\zeta j \in SS$. In the same manner, the key server extracts $TYj \leftarrow H1(IDYj)$ and computes the private key $PVKYj \leftarrow sTYj$, $\forall Yj$ of $\zeta j \in$ SS. Subsequently, the key server sends the private keys PVK_{Xj} and PVK_{Yj} to X_j. Each sender X_j picks n qualified pairs (x'_i, x_i) for $i = 1,..., n$ where $n = |Y_j|$, and computes x $= x'1x'2\cdots x'n$. Then, $\forall \psi 1 \in Yj$, the sender computes a secret key $PVK \psi 1 \leftarrow x_i P-VK_{Yj}$ for $i = 1,..., n$ and distributes $PVK_{\psi 1}$ to ψ_1.

In the Signcrypt algorithm, the sender Xj first signs m by choosing $r \in N*\pi$ and computes $U \leftarrow r_x T_{Xj}$, $\sigma \leftarrow (r_x + H_2 (U \| m)) PVK_{Xj}$ which returns the signature (U, σ). Then, the sender X_j encrypt m using (r, U, σ) for its group members in Y_j to compute

$TYj \leftarrow H1(IDYj)$, $X \leftarrow \gamma (PVKXj, xTYj)$ r, and $W \leftarrow (\sigma \,\|\, IDXj \,\|\, m) \oplus H3(X)$. Then, Xj sends ciphertext (U, W) to its corresponding group members.

For the Unsigncrypt, a member $\psi 1 \in Yj$ decrypts the received ciphertext (U, W) from Xj to compute $Y \leftarrow \gamma (U, PVK\psi 1)$, $\sigma \,\|\, IDXj \,\|\, m \leftarrow W \oplus H3(Y)$. Then, $\psi 1$ computes $T_{Xj} \leftarrow H_1(ID_{Xj})$, $N \leftarrow H_2(U \,\|\, m)$ to verify the signature (U, σ) on message m.

4 Evaluation

In this study, we evaluate the performance of our proposed secure patient information access control scheme by implementing identity-based signcryption into ns-2 simulator. The transport protocol that we used for our simulations is TCP/IP (Transmission Control Protocol/Internet Protocol). The simulation time is set to 100 s. As we perform the simulation, we change the network size to (10, 20, 30, 40, 50, 60) and measure the average time taken to jointly generate the maser private key, the ratio of successful PKG service, and the time taken by the PKG service.

Table 1. Generation time for master key

Network size	Time (s)
10	2.6
20	25.89
30	75.21
40	104.63
50	157.04
60	198.28

Table 1 shows the time for master key generation in terms of different network size. When we increase the network size from 10 to 60, the master key generation time is also increased. This observation can be easily explained as the result of more the transmission delay. To get a master key share, each device needs to get message from any of the n-1 device. As network size becomes larger, the number of transmitted message also became larger which results in a larger transmission delay.

5 Conclusion

The ubiquitous computing environment extends the existing healthcare services provided in medical institutions to the individual and the home. While ubiquitous healthcare introduces great convenience, it also poses at the same time equally great risk.

This paper proposes a secure identity-based signcryption scheme in a network environment. The proposed scheme resolves the sender and data authentication problem by using identity-based signcryption. It also guarantees chosen cipher text security while requiring less performance overhead with regard to the communication, computation, and storage. The identity-based signcryption mechanism is applied here not only to provide end-to-end authenticity and confidentiality in a single step, but also to save network bandwidth and computational power of wireless devices.

Acknowledgment

This paper has been supported by the 2010 Hannam University Research Fund.

References

1. Katsikas, S.K.: Health care management and information systems security: awareness, training or education. Int. J. Med. Informatics 60, 129–135 (2000)
2. Rafaeli, S., Hutchison, D.: A survey of key management for secure group communication. ACM Computing Surveys 35(3), 309–329 (2003)
3. Bohn, J., Gartner, F., Vogt, H.: Dependability Issues of Pervasive Computing in a Health-care Environment. In: Hutter, D., Müller, G., Stephan, W., Ullmann, M. (eds.) Security in Pervasive Computing. LNCS, vol. 2802, pp. 53–70. Springer, Heidelberg (2004), http://www.vs.inf.ethz.ch/res/papers/bohn_pervasivehospital_spc_2003_final.pdf
4. Albrecht, K., McIntyre, L.: Spychips: How Major Corporations and Government Plan to Track Your Every Move with RFID (2005)
5. Weis, S., Sarma, S., Rivest, R., Engels, D.: Security and Privacy Aspects of Low-Cost Radio Frequency Identification Systems. In: Hutter, D., Müller, G., Stephan, W., Ullmann, M. (eds.) Security in Pervasive Computing. LNCS, vol. 2802, pp. 201–212. Springer, Heidelberg (2004)
6. Mavridis, I., Georgiadis, C.K., Pangalos, G., Khair, M.: Using Digital Certificates for Access Control in Clinical Intranet Applications. J. Technol. Health Care 8(3,4), 173–174 (2000)
7. Blundo, C., De Santis, A., Herzberg, A., Kutten, S., Vaccaro, U., Yung, M.: Perfectly-secure key distribution for dynamic conferences. In: Brickell, E.F. (ed.) CRYPTO 1992. LNCS, vol. 740, pp. 471–486. Springer, Heidelberg (1993)
8. Mu, Y., Susilo, W., Lin, W.-X., Ruan, C.: Identity-based authenticated broadcast encryption and distributed authenticated encryption. In: Maher, M.J. (ed.) ASIAN 2004. LNCS, vol. 3321, pp. 169–181. Springer, Heidelberg (2004)
9. Huang, X., Susilo, W., Mu, Y., Zhang, F.: Identity-Based Ring Signcryption Schemes: Cryptographic Primitives for Preserving Privacy and Authenticity in the Ubiquitous World. In: 19th International Conference on Advanced Information Networking and Applications (AINA 2005), vol. 2, pp. 649–654 (2005)
10. Shamir, A.: Identity based cryptosystems and signatures Schemes. In: Blakely, G.R., Chaum, D. (eds.) CRYPTO 1984. LNCS, vol. 196. Springer, Heidelberg (1985)

Towards Improving SCADA Control Systems Security with Vulnerability Analysis

Giovanni Cagalaban and Seoksoo Kim[*]

Department of Multimedia, Hannam University, Ojeong-dong, Daedeok-gu,
306-791 Daejeon, Korea
gcagalaban@yahoo.com, sskim0123@naver.com

Abstract. Cyber security threats and attacks are greatly affecting the security of critical infrastructure, industrial control systems, and Supervisory Control and Data Acquisition (SCADA) control systems. Despite growing awareness of security issues especially in SCADA networks, there exist little or scarce information about SCADA vulnerabilities and attacks. This research addresses the issues regarding security and performs a vulnerability analysis. Modeling of attack trees was created to simulate the vulnerability analysis and carry out assessment methodologies to test existing SCADA security design and implementation. Also, this paper proposes a security framework towards improving security for SCADA control systems.

Keywords: SCADA control system, vulnerability analysis, security framework.

1 Introduction

SCADA networks are composed of control systems that gather data from sensors and instruments located at remote sites and to transmit data at a central site for either control or monitoring purposes [1][2]. With a computer system monitoring and controlling a process which can be industrial, infrastructure or facility-based, many SCADA networks may be susceptible to attacks and misuses because they were developed with little attention being paid to security. Worse, there exist still little or scarce information about SCADA vulnerabilities and attacks, despite the growing awareness of security issues in industrial networks. Even though some vulnerability testing and research are being conducted in this area, very little has been released publicly.

To address the limitations in SCADA security, this study conducts vulnerability assessment methodologies to test the existing SCADA security design and implementation. With the growing concern about the security and safety of the SCADA control systems, this paper provides a relevant analysis of most important issues and a perspective on enhancing security of these systems. This also discusses key developments that mark the evolution of the SCADA control systems along with the increase. Further, this describes key requirements and features needed to improve the security of the current SCADA networks.

---

[*] Corresponding author.

L. Qi (Ed.): PDCN 2010, CCIS 137, pp. 27–32, 2011.

2   Related Works

Various research and assessment activities have revealed an effective methodology for identifying vulnerabilities and developing assessment methods to secure SCADA systems. Applying the probabilistic risk assessment to physical systems was attempted by [3]. Several test tools that have been successful in locating new vulnerabilities in network devices based on grammar and fuzzy techniques are also been developed in academic researches. Considerable work has also been done by [4]. SCADA protocol vulnerabilities, especially the Modbus protocol, were analyzed by Byres [5] and he suggested the use of attack trees to define a series of attacker goals, determine possible means to achieve that goal and identify the weak links of the system. Despite efforts to improve and provide guidance to help ensure program activities address real control system security issues, still there are very little security tools that have been released publicly.

3   SCADA Security Testbed

This research designs a simple prototypical SCADA security testbed to be used for vulnerability assessment. A prototypical SCADA master and slave programs were used to simulate the serial communication between a SCADA master station and RTUs or slaves. Security attacks were simulated using direct access to the infrastructure.

The prototypical security testbed consists of one MTU that communicates with several RTUs. The system used SCADA software for process monitoring and control. RTUs are running a Modbus communication driver to communicate and exchange data with the MTU. We assume that the prototypical SCADA system uses Modbus communication as represented by RS232, RS422 and RS485 communication standard. Modbus protocol was used since it lack inherent security that any moderately skilled hacker would be able to carry out a large variety of attacks if system access can be achieved. Thus, we utilized RS485 and RS232 standards to establish and examine the communication between SCADA Master and RTUs.

3.1   Attack Scenario

In this study, we develop a methodology to illustrate in a structured way the attack possibilities and their relationships. To provide a clear illustration, we design the security testbed and created attack scenarios. One scenario is the man-in-the-middle physical configuration is shown in Fig. 1 wherein the SCADA master and slave is connected with an intruder that sniffs on the network traffic. The man-in-the-middle computer serves as an intruder to perform sniffing and fault injection through the use of a developed program. The goal of this attack was to analyze the communication link between the SCADA communication port and the RTU. Sources of attack can be classified into two types [6]. The first type is internal attacker which comes from the compromised device inside the network. Internal attacks are harder to detect and can potentially create severe damages to the system. Another type of attack is external attack where unauthenticated attackers can steal routing information and inject erroneous information to take control of the system.

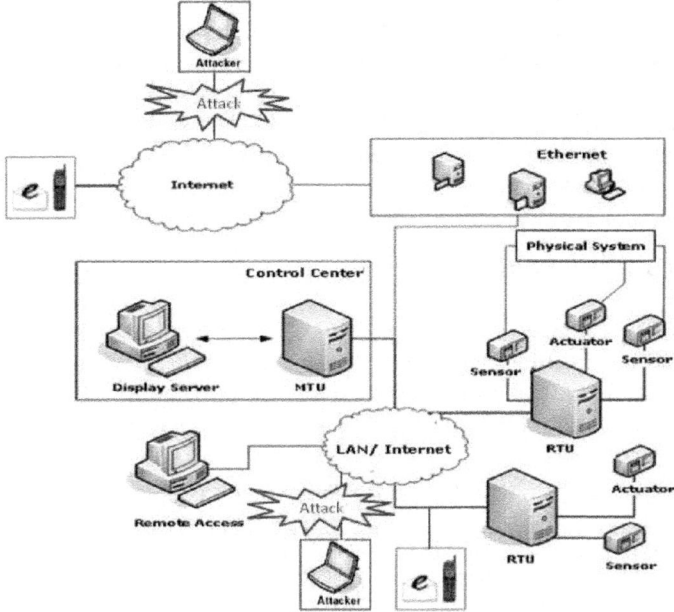

Fig. 1. Sniffing Attack

3.2 Attack Tree Modeling

The use of attack trees as introduced by [7][8] form a convenient way to systematically categorize the different ways in which a system can be attacked. Attack trees are multi-leveled diagrams consisting of one root, leaves, and children.

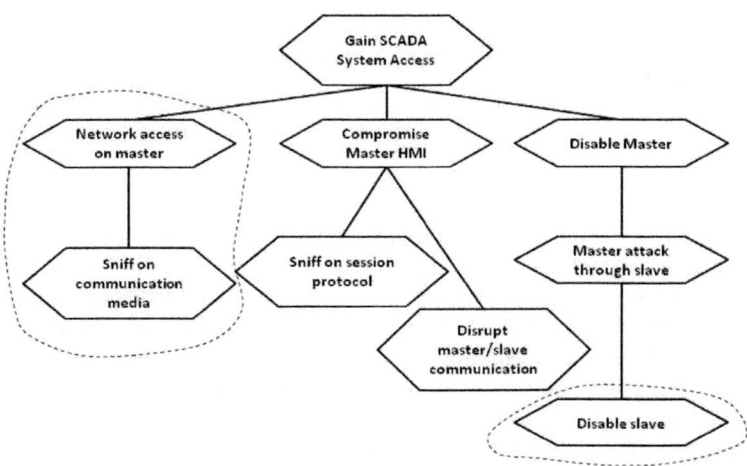

Fig. 2. Attack Tree

To model our attack, we implemented the use of attack trees to provide a more holistic analysis of threats and vulnerabilities and integrating physical, personal, and information security disciplines [9][10]. The graphical and structured tree notation provides us an intuitive aid in our threat analysis process. Using attack trees, we can elaborate events such as specific attack goals in a structured way that must occur for a successful intrusion of the system to take place. Fig. 2 shows an example of an attack tree on the SCADA system.

4   Vulnerability Analysis

To assess the possible security vulnerabilities, some method of assessing and rating the risk of any vulnerability is needed. The impact in this case is an expression of the likelihood that a defined threat will exploit a specific set of vulnerability of a particular attractive target to cause a given set of consequences.

Table 1. Vulnerability Assessment

Attacker's Goal	Attack Type	Impact Rate	Security Recommendation
Gain SCADA system access	Internal	High	Authentication and integrity
Compromise master HMI	Internal	High	Authentication and session
Gain SCADA through remote access	External	Low	Authentication and Transmission media
Network access on master	External	Very Low	Confidentiality and Authentication
Disable master	Internal	Moderate	Authentication and integrity
Master attack through slave	External	Moderate	Frame format and authentication
Disable slave	Internal	Very High	Frame format and authentication

The purpose of the of the analysis is to determine the values associated with the goal of attack to give a better understanding which also reflect the classification of the faults to compromise the whole system. These also indicate where security recommendations are required. Using attack trees allows common attacks to be referenced as reusable modules that apply to multiple network scenarios. Table 1 shows the results of the vulnerability assessment of sniffing activities and compromising the SCADA system.

Vulnerability analysis provides important and critical information for different attack scenarios. For example, these include information such as type and the impact of the attack that would allow an attacker to successfully break the system. Based on the information, the plausibility of each of the attacks can be considered. If one or more attacks are estimated to be likely or possible with improvement in technology over time, the vulnerability analysis would indicate that the current security model must be upgraded or revised.

5   Security Framework

Vulnerability analysis can delineate a security framework that has a potential to guard against the attacks, which are threats to SCADA systems. In this research, vulnerability analysis is presented as effective method for testing SCADA security framework. A method of assessing and rating the risk of any vulnerability is needed. The risk in this case is an expression of the likelihood that a defined threat will exploit a specific set of vulnerability of a particular attractive target to cause a given set of consequences. Fig. 3. shows the proposed security framework. It is a modified version described by Stoneburner [11]. The figure shows an effective calculation of risk which requires a definition of mishap and identification of potential harm to safety. This is calculated as an impact of hazard multiplied by likelihood of mishap event happening.

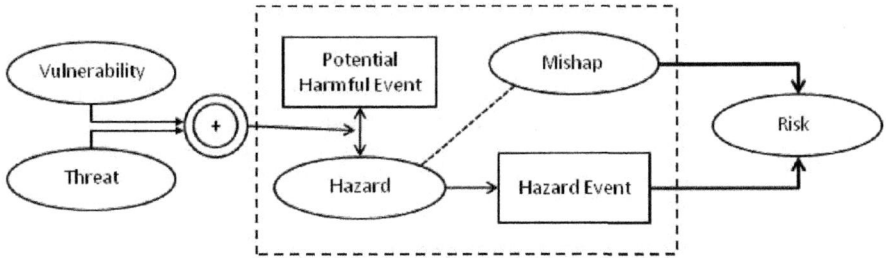

Fig. 3. Security Framework

The effective calculation of risks for SCADA systems bridges the gap between security and safety. With the aid of integrated computer systems, the line that delineates security and safety is almost negligible.

6   Conclusion

The study indicated that the use of these vulnerability assessment in SCADA communications can significantly reduce the vulnerability of these critical systems to malicious cyber attacks, potentially avoiding the serious consequences of such attacks. Implementing security features as those described above ensures higher security, reliability, and availability of control systems. Thus organizations need to reassess the SCADA control systems and risk model to achieve in depth defense solutions for these systems. The increasing threats against SCADA control systems indicate that there should be more directions in the development of these systems. A strategy to deal with cyber attacks against the nation's critical infrastructure requires first understanding the full nature of the threat. A depth defense and proactive solutions to improve the security of SCADA control systems ensures the future of control systems and survivability of critical infrastructure.

References

1. Cepisca, C., Andrei, H., Petrescu, E., Pirvu, C., Petrescu, C.: Remote Data Acquisition System for Hydro Power Plants. In: Proceedings of the 6th WSEAS International Conference on Power Systems, pp. 59–64 (2006)
2. Dobriceanu, M., Bitoleanu, A., Popescu, M., Enache, S., Subtirelu, E.: SCADA System for Monitoring Water Supply Networks. WSEAS Transactions on Systems 1(7), 1070–1079 (2008)
3. Satoh, H., Kumamoto, H.: Viewpoint of ISO GMITS and Probabilistic Risk Assessment in information Security. WSEAS Trans. on Information Science and Application 2, 237–244 (2008)
4. Steven, J.: Adopting an enterprise software security framework. IEEE Security & Privacy 4(2), 84–87 (2006)
5. Byres, E.: Understanding Vulnerabilities in SCADA and Control Systems (2004)
6. Ghaffari, A.: Vulnerability and Security of Mobile Ad hoc Networks. In: Proceedings of the 6th WSEAS International Conference on Simulation, Modelling and Optimization (SMO 2006), pp. 124–129 (2006)
7. Schneier, B.: Attack trees: Modeling security threats. Dr. Dobb's Journal (1999)
8. Khand, P. A.: System Level Security Modeling Using Attack Trees. In: 2nd International Conference on Computer, Control and Communication (IC4 2009), pp. 1-6 (2009)
9. Byres, E., Franz, M., Miller, D.: The use of Attack Trees in Assessing Vulnerabilities in SCADA Systems. In: International Infrastructure Survivability Workshp (IISW). IEEE, Los Alamitos (2004)
10. Poolsapassit, N., Ray, I.: A Systematic Approach for Investigating Computer Attacks Using Attack Trees. In: The 3rd IFIP TC-11 WG 11.9 Working Conference on Digital Forensics (2007)
11. Stoneburner, G.: Toward a unified security/safety model. IEEE Computer 39(8), 96–97 (2006)

Numerical Simulation on Anchorage Effect of Joint Rock

Ning Liu and Chunsheng Zhang

HydroChina, Huadong Engineering Corporation
310014, Hangzhou, China
{liu_n,zhang_cs}@ecidi.com

Abstract. The reinforcement of bolts and shotcrete supporting to rock mass can control the cracks propagation well. Adopt numerical simulation method to study the mechanism of anchorage effect. Use ansys to simulate the effect of bolt to crack. The fore treatment program of crack propagation simulation is compiled by parameterization method of apdl. The calculation and analysis is automatic. Ansys is well for simulating. Analyze the influence of different factors on stress intensity factor. Realize the basic process of fracture analysis in ansys. Prove that bolt plays an important role in control the crack propagation.

Keywords: jointed rock, anchorage effect, ansys, fracture.

1 Introduction

Because there are much jointed cracks and the stress redistribute, there will be more random cracks in surrounding wall after the caverns excavated. The crack generate and propagate, and lead to the surrounding rock damage. Although anchorage has been a successful reinforce treatment, the mechanism is not clear so far. The theory and calculation method is not perfect. The anchorage effect of jointed rock is only depend on numerical method[1].

2 Fracture Analysis Simulation by Ansys

Ansys software provides powerful function and can easily handle before the establishment of the model structure containing defects. The method of mesh guarantees the accuracy is also decrease computing workload of calculation, which is very suitable for contain crack defects or structure. When choosing parameters well, the finite element calculation of the stress intensity factor precision is very good.

The process of ansys fracture analysis can be summarized as follows[2]: (1) the first line around the crack tip is singular element. The unit must be specified at the crack tip for the key point. KSCON commands surrounding the singular element specified points, including 2d unit division arrangement plane183 recommend using 3d unit, use solid95; (2) The slide of main crack surface can be simulated by contact elements; (3) Define the crack tip local coordinate system, require parallel to the crack surface X axis and Y axis perpendicular to crack; (4) Define the path along the crack; (5) Use KCALC command to calculate fracture intensity factor in local coordinate.

L. Qi (Ed.): PDCN 2010, CCIS 137, pp. 33–39, 2011.
© Springer-Verlag Berlin Heidelberg 2011

2.1 Singular Element

The intermediate nodes and unit as to 1/4 position of new unit called singularity unit, it can accurately reflect the crack tip of stress singularities. Singularity unit is a degenerate units, through 8 nodes (2-d) or 20 nodes (3d) element of nodes to 1/4 length to realize, in place of ANSYS help files provided this type of unit, as shown in figure1 and 2.

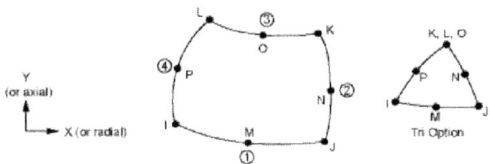

Fig. 1. 2-D singular element

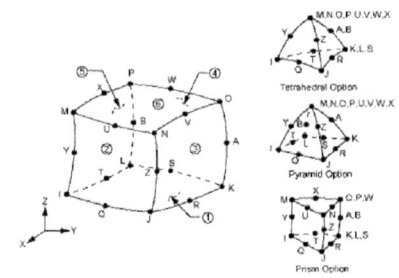

Fig. 2. 3-D singular element

2.2 Contact Analysis

Crack closure pressure fluctuation, crack between surface contact, it will need to use the exposure function analysis software ansys. Ansys support three ways, as point-to-point point-to-surface and surface-surface. For the contact problem, you must realize modeling which parts of the model may contact. Through the contact finite element model is formulated to identify the unit of the contact, may contact elements are covered in the above analysis model of a unit. For 2D contact analysis, considering the crack surface is closed, the contact between the surface. Target and interface with Targe169, Contac172 to simulate a target unit and a contact elements as a contact, through a sharing of program to recognize the real number of often contact.

Usually, the basic steps to establish model and mesh of a surface contact analysis is to identify and target surface contact, definition, define contact, setting unit keyword and constant, define the movement control targets , given the boundary conditions, solve problem solving option, contact, check result.

To sum up, ansys fracture analysis process can be summarized as follows: (1) the first line around the crack tip for the singular element, the unit must be specified at the

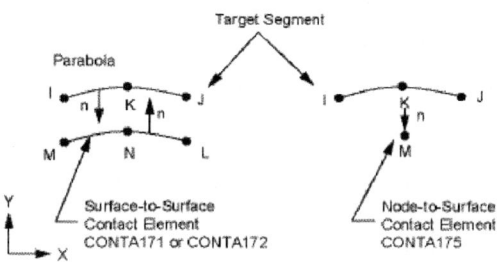

Fig. 3. Targe169 Geometry

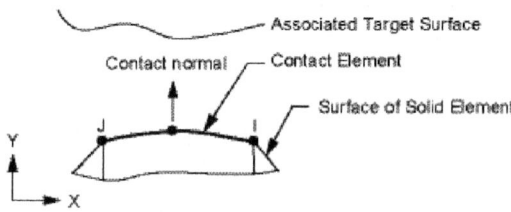

Fig. 4. Contac172 Geometry

crack tip for the key point, KSCON commands surrounding the singular element specified points, including 2d unit division arrangement plane183 recommend using 3d unit, use solid95, 2 the Lord crack with sliding contact elements to simulate, 3 definition of the crack tip local coordinate system, parallel to the crack surface X axis and Y axis perpendicular to crack, 4 the path along the crack definition, 5 KCALC used in local coordinate calculation in command rupture intensity factor.

3   Numerical Analysis on Initiation and Propagation of Wing Crack

3.1   Initiation of Wing Crack

Assume the length of origin crack is 50mm, the dip is 45°, the elastic model is 30GPa, The crack initiation is simulated by ANSYS. From figure.1, there is stress focus in crack tip. The angle between origin crack and wing crack is 70.5°. Combine well with the former results[3].

3.2   Propagation of Wing Crack

Figure.6 is the displacement vector of wing crack tip by ansys. The figure shows that there obvious tension concentration on wing crack tip and lead to crack propagation. All contribute to the wing crack propagation is caused by tension.

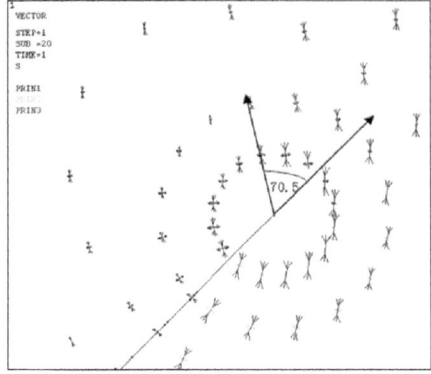 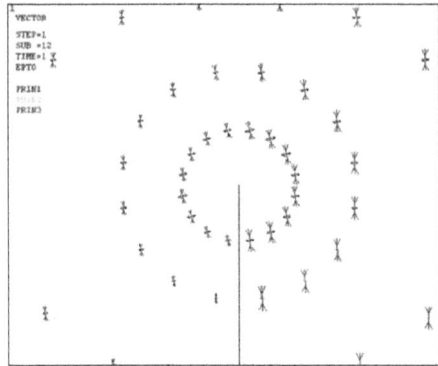

Fig. 5. Vector field of principal stress   **Fig. 6.** Vector field of principal stress

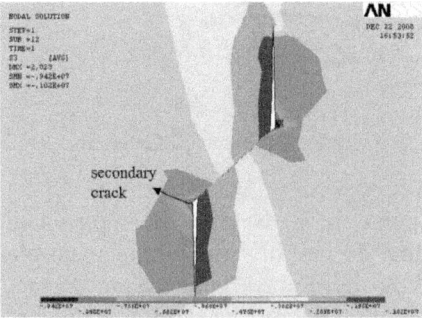

Fig. 7. Distribution of third principal stress of original crack tip

If the wing crack first appeared in the wing crack, after the crack tip of strain accumulation, the part can be released, but the wing cracks formation and propagation, the high compressive stress exists, and crack stress value is very big still. Figure 3 for finite element method to calculate the stress contours of the crack tip, shown in the wing crack formation in the original crack ends after the stress concentration of the phenomenon. With the increase of the load stress concentration, the more obvious phenomenon also, when the shear force than the shear strength, will produce new shear failure, the damage to wing crack with the secondary cracks.

4   Numerical Simulation on Anchorage Effect

Wing crack first from the original crack tip, and craze to the maximum principal stress in the final, so still USES the direction, the numerical model of wing crack model diagram as shown in figure 8. One plane183 unit, still USES rock crack tip, still use KSCON designated as a singular element, the crack tip and the sliding contact with crack, contact element simulation unit. Anchor rod unit link1 unit used. Rock bolting and the interaction between the use of spring unit combin14 unit, with the rock bolting simulation on the connection between each corresponding node using combin14 units 2-d unit to simulate and rock interaction. Ansys help files have the above several units, as shown in figure 9 and 10.

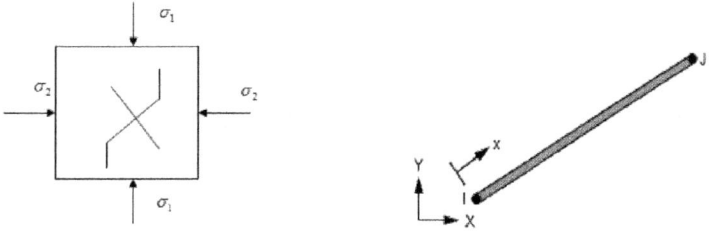

Fig. 8. The sketch of numerical simulation   **Fig. 9.** Bar element of Link1

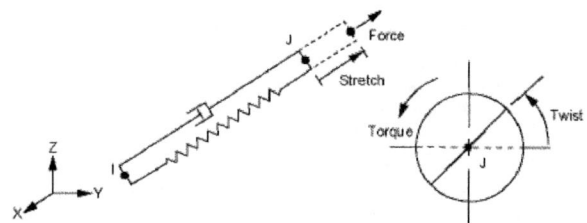

Fig. 10. Spring element of combin14

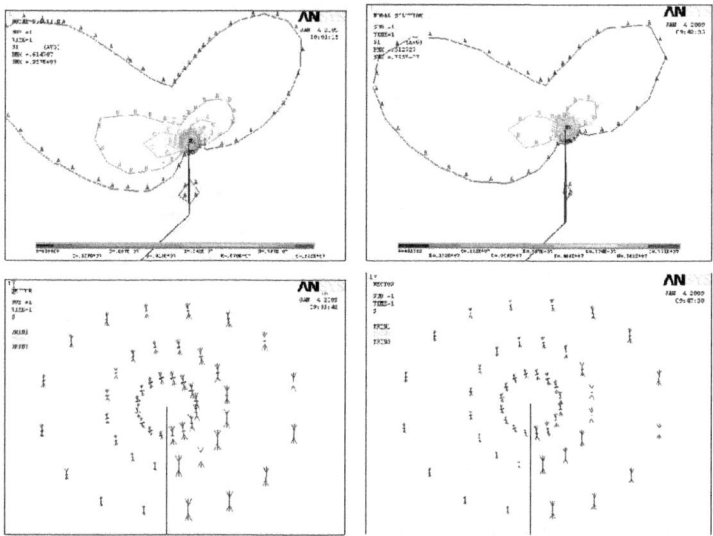

Fig. 11. Contrast of bolted and unbolted

In order to improve the calculation efficiency, especially near the crack wing crack, a step toward the radioactive coarsens. On the surface, the surface under pressure and left for sliding bearing surface, the right side pressure exerted evenly, In the wing crack tip, in order to gain setting singular element calculation results, the ideal around the crack tip, the first line of the unit should be the radius of crack length or smaller.

The results from calculation can be seen at the crack tip, the first principal stress and the principal stress is greatly reduced. But for the maximum principal stress of anchor decreases the minimum principal stress ratio decreased significantly more. But the Lord to crack tip bolt stress direction almost no change, including the wing crack tip and original crack tip, well with the conclusion of figure 12 and 13[4]. When bolted, the crack growth is in need of greater loads, which improve the bearing capacity of the rock.

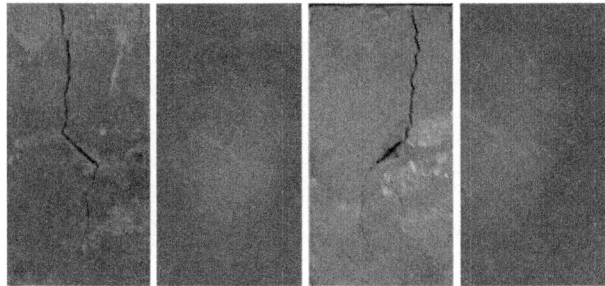

Fig. 12. The finally destroy shape of single crack without bolt

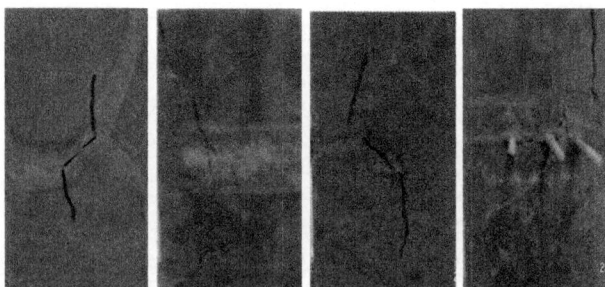

Fig. 13. The finally destroy shape of single crack by bolted middle part

5   Conclusion

Anchorage effect to jointed rock is control the propagation of crack. The paper adopted numerical method to simulate the crack propagation and anchorage effect and achieve good results. Prove that ansys is good for simulating fracture and the bolt plays an important role in restrain the propagation of crack. The numerical result is consist well with the experiment.

References

1. Tang, C.A., Tham, L.G., Lee, P.K.K.: Numerical tests on micro-macro relationship of rock failure under uniaxial compression, part II: constraint, slenderness and size effects. Int. J. Rock Mech. Min. Sci. 37, 570–577 (2000)
2. Nemat-Nasser, S., Obata, M.: A microcrack model of dialatancy in brittle material. J. Appl. Mech. 55, 24–35 (1988)
3. Ravichandran, G., Subhash, G.: A micromechanical model for high strain rate behavior of ceramics. Int. J. Solids Structures 32, 2627–2646 (1995)
4. Hallbauer, D.C., Wagner, H., Cook, N.G.W.: Some observations concerning the microscopic and mechanical behavior of quartzite specimens in stiff, triaxial compressin tests. Int. J. Rock Mech. Min. Sci. 10, 713–725 (1973)

The Judgement for Inverse M-Matrices in Signal Processing

Xueting Liu

School of Electrical and Electronic Engineering, Shandong University of Technology,
Shandong, 255049, People's Republic of China
liuxuet@163.com

Abstract. The inverse M-matrix, as an active research field of matrix, have been applied widely in computational mathematics, economics, biology, physics, numerical computation, signal processing, coding theory, oil investigation in recent years, and so on. In this paper, motivated by [1], we give a simple and convenient judging method, which can be used to judge whether a nonnegative real matrix A is a $n \times n$ inverse M-matrix or not.

Keywords: M-matrix, Inverse M-matrix, Signal Processing.

1 Introduction

The inverse M-matrix, as an active research field of matrix, have been applied widely in computational mathematics, economics, biology, physics, numerical computation, signal processing, coding theory, oil investigation in recent years, and so on.

Nowdays, the properties of inverse M-matrices and their applications are attracting more attention. In [1], GUO Xi-juan,JI Nai-hua,YAO Hui-ping gave a simple and convenient judging methodwhich can be used to judge whether an $n \times n$ nonnegative real matrix A is an inverse M-matrix or not, and reduce the order of an $n \times n$ matrix A gradually until the reduced matrix can be judged by the definition of inverse M-matrices.

In [3], the authors proved that the class of inverse M-matrices is not closed under Hadmard product, and proved that some important subclasses(tridiagonal inverse M-mtrices, Hessenburg inverse M-matrices, and matrices whose inverse are M-matrices with unipathic digraphs) are closed under Hadamard multiplicaiton also. HAN Yin presents three similar structure properties Positive Matrix in the complex number of Inverse M-Matrixes, and one necessary condition for an $n \times n$ Positive Matrix in the complex number field, and concluded the summation Matrix of an arbitrary $n \times n$ Matrix and an inverse M-Matrix is an inverse M-Matrix in [2].

Motivated by the above, especially [1], we give a simple and convenient judging methodwhich can be used to judge whether an $n \times n$ nonnegative real matrix A is an inverse M-matrix or not.

Definition 1.1. Let $Z^{n \times n} = \left\{ A \in R^{n \times n} \middle| a_{ij} \leq 0, i \neq j \right\}$. If $A \in Z^{n \times n}$, then we call A Z-matrix.

L. Qi (Ed.): PDCN 2010, CCIS 137, pp. 40–45, 2011.

Definition 1.2. A matrix $A = [a_{ij}] \in Z^{n \times n}$ is said to be M-matrix, if $A^{-1} \geq 0$.

Definition 1.3. Let $Z^{n \times n} = \{A \in R^{n \times n}\}$ A matrix $A = [a_{ij}] \in Z^{n \times n}$ is said to be positive definite matrix, if for arbitrary $0 \neq x \in R^{n \times 1}$, we have $x^T A x > 0$.

2 Preliminary Notes

In this section, we present some lemmas that are important to our main results.

Lemma 2.1[3, Lemma 6]. Suppose $A = \begin{bmatrix} A_{11} & A_{12} & A_{13} \\ A_{21} & A_{22} & A_{23} \\ A_{31} & A_{32} & A_{33} \end{bmatrix}$, $A = [a_{ij}] \in R^{n \times n}$.

Then A is inverse M-matrix if and only if $A_{11}, H_{22}, H_{33} - H_{32} H_{22}^{-1} H_{23}$ are inverse M-matrices, where

$$H_{22} = A_{22} - A_{21} A_{11}^{-1} A_{12}, H_{32} = A_{32} - A_{31} A_{11}^{-1} A_{12}$$
$$H_{33} = A_{33} - A_{31} A_{11}^{-1} A_{13} H_{23} = A_{23} - A_{21} A_{11}^{-1} A_{13}$$

Lemma 2.2[3, Theorem 1]. Suppose $A = \begin{bmatrix} A_{11} & A_{12} & A_{13} \\ A_{21} & A_{22} & A_{23} \\ A_{31} & A_{32} & A_{33} \end{bmatrix}$, $A = [a_{ij}] \in R^{n \times n}$,

$a_{ij} \leq 0, i \neq j$. Then A is M-matrix if and only if $A_{11}, H_{22}, H_{33} - H_{32} H_{22}^{-1} H_{23}$ are M-matrices, where

$$H_{22} = A_{22} - A_{21} A_{11}^{-1} A_{12}, H_{32} = A_{32} - A_{31} A_{11}^{-1} A_{12}$$
$$H_{33} = A_{33} - A_{31} A_{11}^{-1} A_{13}, H_{23} = A_{23} - A_{21} A_{11}^{-1} A_{13}$$

Lemma 2.3[4]. If $A = [a_{ij}] \in R^{n \times n}$ is M-matrix , then the each principal submatrix of A is M-matrix also.

Lemma 2.4[3, Lemma 2]. Suppose $A = \begin{bmatrix} A_{11} & A_{12} \\ A_{21} & A_{22} \end{bmatrix}$, $A = [a_{ij}] \in R^{n \times n}$. Then A is

inverse M-matrix if and only if $A_{11}, A_{22} - H_{21} H_{11}^{-1} H_{12}$ are inverse M-matrices.

3 The Main Results

In this section, we present our main results.

Theorem 3.1. Suppose $A = \begin{bmatrix} A_{11} & A_{12} & A_{13} & A_{14} \\ A_{21} & A_{22} & A_{23} & A_{24} \\ A_{31} & A_{32} & A_{33} & A_{34} \\ A_{41} & A_{42} & A_{43} & A_{44} \end{bmatrix}$, $A = [a_{ij}] \in R^{n \times n}, a_{ij} > 0$.

Then A is inverse M-matrix if and only if $A_{11}, H_{22}, L_{33}, L_{44} - L_{43}L_{33}^{-1}L_{34}$ are inverse M-matrices, where

$$H_{22} = A_{22} - A_{21}A_{11}^{-1}A_{12}, H_{23} = A_{23} - A_{21}A_{11}^{-1}A_{13},$$
$$H_{24} = A_{24} - A_{21}A_{11}^{-1}A_{14}, H_{32} = A_{32} - A_{31}A_{11}^{-1}A_{12},$$
$$H_{33} = A_{33} - A_{31}A_{11}^{-1}A_{13}, H_{34} = A_{34} - A_{31}A_{11}^{-1}A_{14}$$
$$H_{42} = A_{42} - A_{41}A_{11}^{-1}A_{12}, H_{43} = A_{43} - A_{41}A_{11}^{-1}A_{13},$$
$$H_{44} = A_{44} - A_{41}A_{11}^{-1}A_{14}$$
$$L_{33} = H_{33} - H_{32}H_{22}^{-1}H_{23}, L_{43} = H_{43} - H_{42}H_{22}^{-1}H_{23}$$
$$L_{34} = H_{34} - H_{32}H_{22}^{-1}H_{24}, L_{44} = H_{44} - H_{42}H_{22}^{-1}H_{24}$$

Proof. Let

$$\begin{bmatrix} A_{11} & A_{12} & A_{13} \\ A_{21} & A_{22} & A_{23} \\ A_{31} & A_{32} & A_{33} \end{bmatrix}$$

is inverse M-matrix also. By **Lemma 2.1**, A_{11}, H_{22}, K_{33} are inverse M-matrices. Let

$$C_1 = \begin{bmatrix} I_1 & 0 & 0 & 0 \\ -A_{21}A_{11}^{-1} & I_2 & 0 & 0 \\ -A_{31}A_{11}^{-1} & 0 & I_3 & 0 \\ -A_{41}A_{11}^{-1} & 0 & 0 & I_4 \end{bmatrix}$$

$$C = \begin{bmatrix} I_1 & -A_{21}A_{11}^{-1} & -A_{31}A_{11}^{-1} & -A_{41}A_{11}^{-1} \\ 0 & I_2 & 0 & 0 \\ 0 & 0 & I_3 & 0 \\ 0 & 0 & 0 & I_4 \end{bmatrix}$$

So

$$C_1 AC = \begin{bmatrix} I_1 & 0 & 0 & 0 \\ -A_{21}A_{11}^{-1} & I_2 & 0 & 0 \\ -A_{31}A_{11}^{-1} & 0 & I_3 & 0 \\ -A_{41}A_{11}^{-1} & 0 & 0 & I_4 \end{bmatrix} \begin{bmatrix} A_{11} & A_{12} & A_{13} & A_{14} \\ A_{21} & A_{22} & A_{23} & A_{24} \\ A_{31} & A_{32} & A_{33} & A_{34} \\ A_{41} & A_{42} & A_{43} & A_{44} \end{bmatrix}$$

$$\cdot \begin{bmatrix} I_1 & -A_{21}A_{11}^{-1} & -A_{31}A_{11}^{-1} & -A_{41}A_{11}^{-1} \\ 0 & I_2 & 0 & 0 \\ 0 & 0 & I_3 & 0 \\ 0 & 0 & 0 & I_4 \end{bmatrix}$$

$$= \begin{bmatrix} A_{11} & 0 & 0 & 0 \\ & -A_{21}A_{11}^{-1}A_{12}+A_{22} & -A_{21}A_{11}^{-1}A_{13}+A_{23} & -A_{21}A_{11}^{-1}A_{14}+A_{24} \\ 0 & -A_{31}A_{11}^{-1}A_{12}+A_{32} & -A_{31}A_{11}^{-1}A_{13}+A_{33} & -A_{31}A_{11}^{-1}A_{14}+A_{34} \\ 0 & -A_{41}A_{11}^{-1}A_{12}+A_{42} & -A_{41}A_{11}^{-1}A_{13}+A_{43} & -A_{41}A_{11}^{-1}A_{14}+A_{44} \end{bmatrix}$$

$$= \begin{bmatrix} A_{11} & 0 & 0 & 0 \\ 0 & H_{22} & H_{23} & H_{24} \\ 0 & H_{32} & H_{33} & H_{34} \\ 0 & H_{42} & H_{43} & H_{44} \end{bmatrix}$$

$$= \begin{bmatrix} A_{11} & 0 \\ 0 & A/A_{11} \end{bmatrix} = \begin{bmatrix} A_{11} & 0 \\ 0 & B_1 \end{bmatrix}$$

where

$$H_{22} = A_{22} - A_{21}A_{11}^{-1}A_{12}, H_{23} = A_{23} - A_{21}A_{11}^{-1}A_{13}, H_{24} = A_{24} - A_{21}A_{11}^{-1}A_{14}$$
$$H_{32} = A_{32} - A_{31}A_{11}^{-1}A_{12}, H_{33} = A_{33} - A_{31}A_{11}^{-1}A_{13}, H_{34} = A_{34} - A_{31}A_{11}^{-1}A_{14}$$
$$H_{42} = A_{42} - A_{41}A_{11}^{-1}A_{12}, H_{43} = A_{43} - A_{41}A_{11}^{-1}A_{13}, H_{44} = A_{44} - A_{41}A_{11}^{-1}A_{14}$$

and

$$B_1 = A/A_{11} = \begin{bmatrix} -A_{21}A_{11}^{-1}A_{12}+A_{22} & -A_{21}A_{11}^{-1}A_{13}+A_{23} & -A_{21}A_{11}^{-1}A_{14}+A_{24} \\ -A_{31}A_{11}^{-1}A_{12}+A_{32} & -A_{31}A_{11}^{-1}A_{13}+A_{33} & -A_{31}A_{11}^{-1}A_{14}+A_{34} \\ -A_{41}A_{11}^{-1}A_{12}+A_{42} & -A_{41}A_{11}^{-1}A_{13}+A_{43} & -A_{41}A_{11}^{-1}A_{14}+A_{44} \end{bmatrix}$$

$$= \begin{bmatrix} H_{22} & H_{23} & H_{24} \\ H_{32} & H_{33} & H_{34} \\ H_{42} & H_{43} & H_{44} \end{bmatrix}$$

By **Lemma 2.3**, we know B_1 is inverse M-matrix also. Let

$$L_{33} = H_{33} - H_{32}H_{22}^{-1}H_{23}, L_{43} = H_{43} - H_{42}H_{22}^{-1}H_{23}$$
$$L_{34} = H_{34} - H_{32}H_{22}^{-1}H_{24}, L_{44} = H_{44} - H_{42}H_{22}^{-1}H_{24}$$

By **Lemma 2.2**, $L_{33}, H_{44} - H_{43}H_{33}^{-1}H_{34}$ are inverse M-matriced.

We shall show the sufficiency. if $A_{11}, H_{22}, K_{33}, K_{44} - K_{43}K_{33}^{-1}K_{34}$ are inverse M-matrices,

$$A_{11}^{-1}, H_{22}^{-1}, K_{33}^{-1}, \left(K_{44} - K_{43}K_{33}^{-1}K_{34} \right)^{-1}$$

are M-matrices. Due to

$$K_1^{-1} = P \begin{bmatrix} K_{33}^{-1} & 0 \\ 0 & \left(K_{44} - K_{43}K_{33}^{-1}K_{34} \right)^{-1} \end{bmatrix} P_1,$$

$$a_{ij} \geq 0, \ K_{33}^{-1}, \left(K_{44} - K_{43}K_{33}^{-1}K_{34} \right)^{-1}$$

are M-matrices and the constitution of P_1, P, it's easy to see that the off-diagonal elements of K_1^{-1} are not positive numbers, by **Lemma 2.4**, K_1^{-1} is M-matrix.Considering

$$B_1^{-1} = D \begin{bmatrix} H_{22}^{-1} & 0 \\ 0 & K_1^{-1} \end{bmatrix} D_1,$$

for the same reason, the off-diagonal elements of B_1^{-1} are not positive numbers, by **Lemma 2.4**, B_1^{-1} is M-matrix. Since

$$A^{-1} = C \begin{bmatrix} A_{11}^{-1} & 0 \\ 0 & B_1^{-1} \end{bmatrix} C_1,$$

the off-diagonal elements of A^{-1} are not positive numbers also. In addition, $\left(A^{-1} \right)^{-1} = A \geq 0$. By the definition, A^{-1} is M-matrix. So A is inverse M-matrix. This completes the proof.

References

[1] Guo, X.-j., Ji, N.-h., Yao, H.-p.: The Judgement and Parallel Algorithm for Inverse M-matrixes. Journal of Beihua University 45, 97–103 (2004)

[2] Han, Y.: The Property and Judgment of Inverse M-Matrixes. Journal of Huzhou Teachers College 30, 10–12 (2008)

[3] Yang, C.-s., Yang, S.-j.: Closure Properties of Inverse M-matrices under Hadamard Product. Journal of Anhui University(Natural Sciences) 4, 15–20 (2000)

[4] Yang, z.-y., Fu, Y.-d., Huang, T.-z.: Some Properties of InverseM-Matrices and Their Applications. Joumal of UEST of China 34, 713–716 (2005)

[5] Lou, X.-y., Cui, B.-t.: Exponential dissipativity of Cohen-Grossberg neural networks with mixed delays and reaction-diffusion terms 4, 619–922 (2008)

[6] You, Z.: Nonsingular M-matrix. Huazhong University of Science and Technology Publishing House, Wuhan (1983)

[7] Zhaolin, J.: Non singularity on scaled factor circulant matrices. Journal of Baoji College of Arts and Science (Natural Science) 23, 5–7 (2003)

[8] Cline, R.E., Plemmons, R.J., Worm, G.: Generalized inverses of certain Toeplitz matrices. Linear Algebra and Its Applications 8, 25–33 (1974)

[9] Zhaolin, J.: Non singularity on r-circulant matrices. Mathematics in Practice and Theory 2, 52–58 (1995)

[10] Li, H., Liu, X., Zhao, W.: Nonsingularity on Scaled Factor Circulant Matrices. International Journal of Algebra 2(18), 889–893 (2008)

[11] Jiang, J.: Two Simple Methods of Finding Inverse Matrix of Cyclic Matrix. Journal of Jiangxi Institute of Education(Comprehensive) 3, 5–6 (2008)

[12] Deng, Y.: Problem of Cyclic Matrix Inversion. Journal of Hengyang Normal University 3, 31–33 (1995)

[13] Lai, Y., Chen, Y., Zheng, R.: The fast Fourier transform algorithm for the production of the permutation factor circulant matrices. Journal of Baoji University of Arts and Sciences (Natural Science) 24(4), 262–264 (2008)

[14] Zhaolin, J., Zhou, Z.: Circulant Matrices. Chengdu Technology University Publishing Company, Chengdu (1999)

[15] Shen, G.: The Time Complexity of r-circulant Syestems. Journal Mathematical Research and Exposition 4, 595–598 (1992)

[16] Zhaolin, J., Liu, S.: The Fast Algorithm for Finding the Inverse and Generalized Inverse of Permutation Factor Circulant Matrix. Numerical Mathematics A Journal of Chinese Universities 03, 227–234 (2003)

Estimates for the Upper and Lower Bounds on the Inverse Elements of Strictly Diagonally Dominant Periodic Adding Element Tridiagonal Matrices in Signal Processing

Wenling Zhao

College of Science Shandong University of Technology
Shandong, 255049, People's Republic of China
zwlsdj@163.com

Abstract. Strictly diagonally dominant periodic adding element tridiagonal matrices play a very important role in the theory and practical applications. In this paper, Motivated by the references, especially [2], we give the estimates for the upper bounds on the inverse elements of strictly diagonally dominant periodic adding element tridiagonal matrices.

Keywords: strictly diagonally dominant, Adding Element Tridiagonal Matrices, inverse matrix, Signal Processing, upper bounds.

1 Introduction

Tridiagonal matrices have been widely applied in signal processing, economics, physics, in recent years, and so on. To solve tridiagonal linear systems using parallel computers, and also to derive bounds for the inverse of finite and infinite tridiagonal matrices, many algorithms have been studied Such as in [2], [3], [4], [5], [6], [7].

Motivated by the above, especially [2], we give the upper bounds for inverse elements of strictly diagonally dominant periodic adding element tridiagonal matrices.

Definition 1.1. A matrix $A = [a_{ij}] \in Z^{n \times n}$ is said to be tridiagonal period matrix, if A has the form

$$
\begin{pmatrix}
a_1 & b_1 & 0 & \cdots & & d_1 \\
c_1 & a_2 & b_2 & \ddots & & \vdots \\
0 & c_2 & a_3 & \ddots & & 0 \\
\vdots & \ddots & \ddots & \ddots & & b_{n-1} \\
d_2 & \cdots & & 0 & c_{n-1} & a_n
\end{pmatrix}
\tag{1}
$$

Definition 1.2. A matrix $A = [a_{ij}] \in Z^{n \times n}$ is said to be adding element tridiagonal period matrix, if it has the form

L. Qi (Ed.): PDCN 2010, CCIS 137, pp. 46–51, 2011.

$$\begin{pmatrix} a_1 & b_1 & 0 & d_1 & 0 & \vdots & 0 & d_2 \\ c_1 & a_2 & b_2 & 0 & 0 & \ddots & 0 & 0 \\ 0 & c_2 & a_3 & b_3 & 0 & \ddots & 0 & 0 \\ e_1 & 0 & c_3 & a_4 & b_4 & \ddots & 0 & 0 \\ 0 & 0 & 0 & c_4 & a_5 & \ddots & 0 & 0 \\ \vdots & \ddots & \ddots & \ddots & \ddots & \ddots & \ddots & \vdots \\ 0 & \cdots & 0 & 0 & 0 & c_{n-1} & a_{n-1} & b_{n-1} \\ e_2 & \cdots & 0 & 0 & 0 & 0 & c_{n-1} & a_n \end{pmatrix} \tag{2}$$

For simplicity, in this paper, we note the tridiagonal matrix

$$T = \begin{pmatrix} a_1 & b_1 & 0 & \cdots & 0 \\ c_1 & a_2 & b_2 & \ddots & \vdots \\ 0 & c_2 & a_3 & \ddots & 0 \\ \vdots & \ddots & \ddots & \ddots & b_{n-1} \\ 0 & \cdots & 0 & c_{n-1} & a_n \end{pmatrix}$$

by $tri(a_i,c_i,b_i)_{i=1}^n$, note the tridiagonal period matrix by $tri(a_i,c_i,b_i,d_1,d_2)_{i=1}^n$, and note the adding element tridiagonal period matrix by $tri(a_i,c_i,b_i,d_1,d_2,e_1,e_2)_{i=1}^n$.

Definition 1.3. A matrix $A=[a_{ij}]\in Z^{n\times n}$ is said to be strictly diagonally dominant periodic adding element tridiagonal matrix, if A is row diagonally dominant, i.e.,

$$|a_1|>|b_1|+|d_1|+|d_2|, |a_2|>|c_1|+|b_2|,$$
$$|a_3|>|c_2|+|b_3|, |a_4|>|e_1|+|c_3|+|b_4|,$$
$$|a_5|>|c_4|+|b_5|,\cdots,|a_{n-1}|>|c_{n-1}|+|b_{n-1}|,$$
$$|a_n|>|e_1|+|c_{n-1}|$$

2 Preliminary Notes

In this section, we present some lemmas that are important to our main results.

Lemma 2.1[10]. Let (1) be partitioned as

$$A = \begin{pmatrix} T_1 & \alpha \\ \beta^T & a_n \end{pmatrix} = \begin{pmatrix} a_1 & \hat{\beta}^T \\ \hat{\alpha} & T_2 \end{pmatrix}$$

where

$$T_1 = tri(a_i,c_i,b_i)_{i=1}^{n-1}, T_2 = tri(a_i,c_i,b_i)_{i=2}^{n},$$

$$\alpha = \begin{pmatrix} d_1 \\ 0 \\ \vdots \\ 0 \\ b_{n-1} \end{pmatrix}, \beta = \begin{pmatrix} d_2 \\ 0 \\ \vdots \\ 0 \\ c_{n-1} \end{pmatrix}, \hat{\beta} = \begin{pmatrix} b_1 \\ 0 \\ \vdots \\ 0 \\ d_1 \end{pmatrix} \hat{\alpha} = \begin{pmatrix} c_1 \\ 0 \\ \vdots \\ 0 \\ d_2 \end{pmatrix}$$

If A, T_1, T_2 are nonsingular, then

$$\omega = a_n - \beta^T T_1^{-1}\alpha \neq 0, \hat{\omega} = a_1 - \hat{\beta}^T T_2^{-1}\hat{\alpha} \neq 0$$

and

$$A^{-1} = \begin{pmatrix} T_1^{-1} + \dfrac{T_1^{-1}\alpha\beta^T T_1^{-1}}{\omega} & -\dfrac{T_1^{-1}\alpha}{\omega} \\ -\dfrac{\beta^T T_1^{-1}}{\omega} & \dfrac{1}{\omega} \end{pmatrix} = \begin{pmatrix} \dfrac{1}{\hat{\omega}} & -\dfrac{\hat{\beta}^T T_2^{-1}}{\hat{\omega}} \\ -\dfrac{T_2^{-1}\hat{\alpha}}{\hat{\omega}} & T_2^{-1} + \dfrac{T_2^{-1}\hat{\alpha}\hat{\beta}^T T_2^{-1}}{\hat{\omega}} \end{pmatrix}$$

Lemma 2.2[2, Theorem 2.1]. Suppose tridiagonal matrix $T = tri(a_i,c_i,b_i)_{i=1}^{n}$ is strictly diagonally dominant according to row, i. e. satisfy

$$|a_1| > |b_1|, |a_i| > |c_{i-1}| + |b_i|(i = 2,\cdots,n), |a_n| > |c_{n-1}|,$$

and $b_i c_i \neq 0 (i = 1,2,\cdots,n-1)$. Let $\{w_i\}, \{r_i\}$ be the elements in the first row and in the last row of T^{-1}, that is

$$\mu = (u_1,u_2,\cdots,u_n) = e_1^T T^{-1}, v = (v_1,v_2,\cdots,v_n) = e_n^T T^{-1}$$

then we have

$$|u_1| \leq \frac{1}{|a_1| - \omega_2|b_1|}, |u_k| \leq \frac{|b_{k-1}|\omega_k}{|c_{k-1}|} (k = 2,\cdots,n)$$

$$|v_n| \leq \frac{1}{|a_n| - \tau_{n-1}|c_{n-1}|}, |v_k| \leq \frac{|c_k|\tau_k}{|b_k|} (k = n-1,\cdots,1)$$

where

$$\tau_1 = \frac{|b_1|}{|a_1|}, \tau_i = \frac{|b_i|}{|a_i| - |c_{i-1}|}(i = 2, \cdots, n-1)$$

$$\omega_n = \frac{|c_{n-1}|}{|a_n|}, \omega_i = \frac{|c_{i-1}|}{|a_i| - |b_i|}(i = n-1, \cdots, 2)$$

Lemma 2.3[3]. If $A \in R^{n \times n}$ is strictly diagonally dominant according to row, then A^{-1} is strictly diagonally dominant according to column, namely , if $A^{-1} = (v_{ij})_{n \times n}$, then $|v_{ii}| > |v_{ji}| (j \neq i)$.

3 The Main Results

In this section, we present our main results.

Theorem 3.1. If the tridiagonal period matrix $A = tri(a_i, c_i, b_i, d_1, d_2)_{i=1}^n$ is strictly diagonally dominant according to row. Let $A^{-1} = (v_{ij})_{n \times n}$, then

$$|v_{ii}| \geq \frac{1}{|a_i| + |b_i| + |c_i|}(i \neq 1, n)$$

$$|v_{11}| \geq \frac{1}{|a_1| + |b_1| + |d_2|}$$

$$|v_{nn}| \geq \frac{1}{|d_1| + |c_{n-1}| + |a_n|}$$

Proof. The proof is similarly to [2, **Theorem 2.2**]

Since $A = tri(a_i, c_i, b_i, d_1, d_2)_{i=1}^n$ is row strictly diagonally dominant, it is easy to see

$$\det A, M_i, N_i, P_i \neq 0$$

By *Cramer's* rule, we have

$$v_{ii} = \frac{N_i}{\det A} = \frac{N_i}{-c_{i-1}M_i + a_i N_i - b_i P_i}$$

$$= \frac{1}{-c_{i-1}\dfrac{M_i}{N_i} + a_i - b_i \dfrac{P_i}{N_i}}(i \neq 1, n)$$

where M_i, N_i, P_i are the cofactor of c_{i-1}, a_i, b_i respectively. By Lemma 2.3, A^{-1} is strictly diagonally dominant according to column, so

$$\frac{|M_i|}{|N_i|} < 1, \frac{|P_i|}{|N_i|} < 1$$

Hence

$$\left| -c_{i-1}\frac{M_i}{N_i} + a_i - b_i \frac{P_i}{N_i} \right| \leq |a_i| + |b_i| + |c_i|$$

So

$$|v_{ii}| \geq \frac{1}{|a_i| + |b_i| + |c_i|}(i \neq 1, n)$$

Similarly, we can proof

$$|v_{11}| \geq \frac{1}{|a_1| + |b_1| + |d_2|}$$

$$|v_{nn}| \geq \frac{1}{|d_1| + |c_{n-1}| + |a_n|}$$

This completes the proof.

References

[1] Zhu, H.: The Criteria Of Specific Shape Invers M– Matrices, Xiangtan University Master's Thesis (2007)
[2] Yuan, Z.-j.: The Research on the Computing Problems and the Properties about Special Matrices, Northwestern Polytechnical University Master's Thesis (2005)
[3] Chen, J., Chen, X.: Special Matrix. Tsinghua University Press, Beijing (2001)
[4] Xu, Z.: Upper Bounds for Inverse Elements of Strictly Diagonally Dominant Periodic Tridiagonal Matrices. Chinese Journal of Engineering Mathematics 21, 67–72 (2004)
[5] Peluso, R., Politi, T.: Some improvements for two-sided bounds on the inverse of diagonally dominant tridiagonal matrices. Linear. Algebr. Appl. 330, 1–14 (2001)
[6] Liu, X., Huang, T., Fu, Y.-D.: Estimates for the inverse elements of tridiagonal matrices. Applied Mathematics Letters 194, 590–598 (2006)
[7] Kershaw, D.: Inequalities on the elements of the inverse of a certain tridiagonal matrix. Math. Comput. 24, 155–158 (1970)

[8] Nabben, R.: Two-sided bounds on the inverse of diagonally dominant tridiagonal matrices. Linear Algebr. Appl. 287, 289–305 (1999)

[9] Yang, C.-s., Yang, S.-j.: Closure Properties of Inverse M-matrices under Hadamard Product. Journal of Anhui University(Natural Sciences) 4, 15–20 (2000)

[10] Xiu, Z., Zhang, K., Lu, Q.: Fast algorithm for Toeplitz matrix. Northwestern Polytechnical University Press (1999)

[11] Lou, X.-y., Cui, B.-t.: Exponential dissipativity of Cohen-Grossberg neural networks with mixed delays and reaction-diffusion terms 4, 619–922 (2008)

[12] Guo, X.-j., Ji, N.-h., Yao, H.-p.: The Judgement and Parallel Algorithm for Inverse M-matrixes. Journal of Beihua University 45, 97–103 (2004)

[13] Yang, z.-y., Fu, Y.-d., Huang, T.-z.: Some Properties of InverseM-Matrices and Their Applications. Journal of UEST of China 34, 713–716 (2005)

[14] Han, Y.: The Property and Judgment of Inverse M-Matrixes. Journal of Huzhou Teachers College 30, 10–12 (2008)

[15] You, Z.: Nonsingular M-matrix. Huazhong University of Science and Technology Publishing House, Wuhan (1983)

[16] Zhaolin, J.: Non singularity on scaled factor circulant matrices. Journal of Baoji College of Arts and Science (Natural Science) 23, 5–7 (2003)

[17] Li, H., Liu, X., Zhao, W.: Nonsingularity on Scaled Factor Circulant Matrices. International Journal of Algebra 2(18), 889–893 (2008)

[18] Zhaolin, J.: Non singularity on r-circulant matrices. Mathematics in Practice and Theory 2, 52–58 (1995)

[19] Deng, Y.: Problem of Cyclic Matrix Inversion. Journal of Hengyang Normal University 3, 31–33 (1995)

[20] Jiang, J.: Two Simple Methods of Finding Inverse Matrix of Cyclic Matrix. Journal of Jiangxi Institute of Education(Comprehensive) 3, 5–6 (2008)

A Fast Algorithm for the Inverse Matrices of Periodic Adding Element Tridiagonal Matrices

Hongkui Li and Ranran Li

College of Science Shandong University of Technology
Shandong, 255049, People's Republic of China
lhk8068@163.com, liranran_1213@qq.com

Abstract. Adding element tridiagonal periodic matrices have an important effect for the algorithms of solving linear systems, computing the inverses, the triangular factorization, the boundary value problems by finite difference methods, interpolation by cubic splines, three-term difference equations and so on. In this paper, we give a fast algorithm for the Inverse Matrices of periodic adding element tridiagonal matrices.

Keywords: Tridiagonal Matrices, Periodic Tridiagonal Matrices, Periodic Adding Element Tridiagonal Matrices, inverse matrix.

1 Introduction

Solving linear systems, computing the inverses and the triangular factorization have extensive application in signal processing, economics, physics, biology, numerical computation, coding theory, computational mathematics, applied mathematics, oil investigation in recent years, and so on. On many conditions, however, the solving of linear systems, the computing the inverses and the triangular factorization usually need special matrices. As one kind of them, Tridiagonal matrices arise in many topics of numerical analysis including the boundary value problems by finite difference methods, interpolation by cubic splines, three-term difference equations and so on. They play an important role more and more. Therefore it can give improvements by great progress obtained in the researches on special matrices in computational mathematics.

Many algorithms have been studied to solve tridiagonal linear systems using parallel computers,and also to derive bounds for the inverse of finite and infinite tridiagonal matrices[3]such as in [3], YUAN Zhi-jie, XU Zhong gave the upper bounds for inverse elements of strictly diagonally dominant periodic tridiagonal matrices. In [4], the authors gave easily computable upper and lower bounds for the inverse elements of finite tridiagonal diagonally dominant matrices,and we improve the well-known upper bounds due to Ostrowski.

In this paper, motivated by the above, especially[3], we give a fast algorithm for the Inverse Matrices of periodic adding element tridiagonal matrices.

L. Qi (Ed.): PDCN 2010, CCIS 137, pp. 52–57, 2011.
© Springer-Verlag Berlin Heidelberg 2011

Definition 1.1. A matrix $A = [a_{ij}] \in Z^{n \times n}$ is said to be tridiagonal period matrix, if A has the form

$$
\begin{pmatrix}
a_1 & b_1 & 0 & \cdots & & & d_1 \\
c_1 & a_2 & b_2 & \ddots & & & \vdots \\
0 & c_2 & a_3 & \ddots & & & 0 \\
\vdots & \ddots & \ddots & \ddots & & b_{n-1} \\
d_2 & \cdots & & 0 & c_{n-1} & a_n
\end{pmatrix} = tri(a_i, c_i, b_i, d_1, d_2)_{i=1}^n \tag{1}
$$

Definition 1.2. A matrix $A = [a_{ij}] \in Z^{n \times n}$ is said to be adding element tridiagonal period matrix, if it has the form

$$
\begin{pmatrix}
a_1 & b_1 & 0 & d_1 & 0 & \vdots & 0 & d_2 \\
c_1 & a_2 & b_2 & 0 & 0 & \ddots & 0 & 0 \\
0 & c_2 & a_3 & b_3 & 0 & \ddots & 0 & 0 \\
e_1 & 0 & c_3 & a_4 & b_4 & \ddots & 0 & 0 \\
0 & 0 & 0 & c_4 & a_5 & \ddots & 0 & 0 \\
\vdots & \ddots & \ddots & \ddots & \ddots & \ddots & \ddots & \vdots \\
0 & \cdots & 0 & 0 & 0 & c_{n-2} & a_{n-1} & b_{n-1} \\
e_2 & \cdots & 0 & 0 & 0 & 0 & c_{n-1} & a_n
\end{pmatrix} = tri(a_i, c_i, b_i, d_1, d_2, e_1, e_2)_{i=1}^n \tag{2}
$$

2 Preliminary Notes

In this section, we present some lemmas that are important to our main results.

Lemma 2.1[2]. If the tridiagonal matrix $tri(b_i, a_i, c_i)_{i=1}^n$ is nonsingular, and $b_i c_i \neq 0 (i = 1, 2, \cdots, n-1)$. Let $\{u_i\}, \{v_i\}$ be the elements in the first row and in the last row of A^{-1}, that is

$$
\mu = \begin{pmatrix} u_1 & u_2 & \cdots & u_n \end{pmatrix} = e_1^T A^{-1}, v = \begin{pmatrix} v_1 & v_2 & \cdots & v_n \end{pmatrix} = e_n^T A^{-1}
$$

Then we can calculate $\{u_i\}, \{v_i\}$ by the recursive formula

$$
\begin{cases}
d_n = b_n, d_i = b_i - \dfrac{a_i c_i}{d_{i+1}}(i = n-1,\cdots,1) \\[2mm]
u_1 = \dfrac{1}{d_1}, u_k = -\dfrac{c_{k+1}}{d_k}u_{k-1}(k = 2,\cdots,n) \\[2mm]
\delta_1 = b_1, \delta_i = b_i - \dfrac{a_{i-1}c_{i-1}}{\delta_{i-1}}(i = 2,\cdots,n) \\[2mm]
v_n = \dfrac{1}{\delta_n}, v_k = -\dfrac{a_k}{\delta_k}v_{k+1}(k = n-1,\cdots,1)
\end{cases}
$$

Lemma 2.2[8]. Let (1) be partitioned as

$$
A = \begin{pmatrix} T_1 & \alpha \\ \beta^T & a_n \end{pmatrix} = \begin{pmatrix} a_1 & \hat{\beta}^T \\ \hat{\alpha} & T_2 \end{pmatrix},
$$

where

$$
T_1 = tri(a_i, c_i, b_i)_{i=1}^{n-1}, T_2 = tri(a_i, c_i, b_i)_{i=2}^{n},
$$

$$
\alpha = \begin{pmatrix} d_1 \\ 0 \\ \vdots \\ 0 \\ b_{n-1} \end{pmatrix}, \beta = \begin{pmatrix} d_2 \\ 0 \\ \vdots \\ 0 \\ c_{n-1} \end{pmatrix}, \hat{\beta} = \begin{pmatrix} b_1 \\ 0 \\ \vdots \\ 0 \\ d_1 \end{pmatrix} \hat{\alpha} = \begin{pmatrix} c_1 \\ 0 \\ \vdots \\ 0 \\ d_2 \end{pmatrix}
$$

If A, T_1, T_2 are nonsingular, then

$$
\omega = a_n - \beta^T T_1^{-1}\alpha \neq 0, \hat{\omega} = a_1 - \hat{\beta}^T T_2^{-1}\hat{\alpha} \neq 0
$$

and

$$
A^{-1} = \begin{pmatrix} T_1^{-1} + \dfrac{T_1^{-1}\alpha\beta^T T_1^{-1}}{\omega} & -\dfrac{T_1^{-1}\alpha}{\omega} \\[3mm] -\dfrac{\beta^T T_1^{-1}}{\omega} & \dfrac{1}{\omega} \end{pmatrix} = \begin{pmatrix} \dfrac{1}{\hat{\omega}} & -\dfrac{\hat{\beta}^T T_2^{-1}}{\hat{\omega}} \\[3mm] -\dfrac{T_2^{-1}\hat{\alpha}}{\hat{\omega}} & T_2^{-1} + \dfrac{T_2^{-1}\hat{\alpha}\hat{\beta}^T T_2^{-1}}{\hat{\omega}} \end{pmatrix}
$$

3 The Main Results

In this section, we present our main results.

Theorem. If the adding element tridiagonal period matrix $tri(a_i, c_i, b_i, d_1, d_2, e_1, e_2)_{i=1}^n$ is nonsingular, and $b_i c_i \neq 0 (i = 1, 2, \cdots, n-1)$. Let $A^{-1} = (v_{ij})_{n \times n}$, then there are sequence $\{u_i\}, \{v_i\}$ $\{w_i\}, \{r_i\}$, such that

$$
\begin{cases}
v_{3,j} = -\dfrac{\dfrac{1}{c_3} e_1 + (a_4 w_4 + b_4 w_5)}{c_3} u_j - \dfrac{(a_4 r_4 + b_4 r_5)}{c_3} v_j, (j = 1, 2, 3) \\
v_{i-1,j} = w_{i-1} u_j + r_{i-1} v_j, (i > j+1, i \neq 4, j \neq 1, 2, 3)
\end{cases}
$$

Proof. Let $\{w_i\}, \{r_i\}$ be the elements in the first row and in the last row of A^{-1}, that is

$$
\mu = (u_1 \quad u_2 \quad \cdots \quad u_n) = e_1^T A^{-1}, v = (v_1 \quad v_2 \quad \cdots \quad v_n) = e_n^T A^{-1}
$$

Since $AA^{-1} = I_n$, by

$$
c_1 u_j + a_2 v_{2,j} + b_2 v_j = 0, (j < n)
$$

We have

$$
v_{2,j} = -\frac{c_1}{a_2} u_j - \frac{b_2}{a_2} v_j = w_2 u_j + r_2 v_j, (j < n)
$$

where

$$
w_2 = -\frac{c_1}{a_2} u_j, r_2 = -\frac{b_2}{a_2} \tag{3.1}
$$

If $v_{i,j} = w_2 u_j + r_2 v_j, (i > j)$, by
$c_{i-1} v_{i-1,j} + a_i v_{ij} + b_i v_{i+1,j} = 0, (i+1 \leq j, i \neq 4, j \neq 1, 2, 3)$, we have

$$
(a_i w_i + b_i w_{i+1}) u_j + (c_i r_i + a_i r_{i+1}) v_j + b_{i-1} v_{i-1,j} = 0
$$

Therefore,

$$
v_{i-1,j} = w_{i-1} u_j + r_{i-1} v_j, (i > j+1, i \neq 4, j \neq 1, 2, 3)
$$

where

$$
w_{i-1} = -\frac{(a_i w_i + b_i w_{i+1})}{b_{i-1}} u_j, r_{i-1} = -\frac{(c_i r_i + a_i r_{i+1})}{b_{i-1}} (i = 2, 3, \cdots, n-2, i \neq 4) \tag{3.2}
$$

If $v_{i,j} = w_2 u_j + r_2 v_j, (i \leq j)$ and $i = 4$, by
$e_1 u_j + c_3 v_{3,j} + a_4 v_{4,j} + b_4 v_{5,j} = 0, (5 \leq j)$ and (3.2), we have

$$e_1 u_j + c_3 v_{3,j} + a_4 (w_4 u_j + r_4 v_j) + b_4 (w_5 u_j + r_5 v_j) = 0,$$

Hence,

$$v_{3,j} = -\frac{\dfrac{1}{c_3} e_1 + (a_4 w_4 + b_4 w_5)}{c_3} u_j - \frac{(a_4 r_4 + b_4 r_5)}{c_3} v_j, \qquad (3.3)$$

Let

$$w_1 = 1, r_1 = 0, w_n = 0, r_n = 1 \qquad (3.4)$$

By (3.1) (3.2) (3.3) and (3.4), we can calculate $\{u_i\}, \{v_i\}$

This completes the proof.

References

[1] Shivakumar, P.N., Ji, C.: Upper and lower bounds for inverse elements of finite and infinite tridiagonal matrices. Linear Algebra Appl. 247, 297–316 (1996)

[2] Yuan, Z.-j., Xu, Z.: Upper Bounds for Inverse Elements of Strictly Diagonally Dominant Periodic Tridiagonal Matrices. Chinese Journal of Engineering Mathematics 21, 67–72 (2004)

[3] Peluso, R., Politi, T.: Some improvements for two-sided bounds on the inverse of diagonally dominant tridiagonal matrices. Linear. Algebr. Appl. 330, 1–14 (2001)

[4] Liu, X., Huang, T., Fu, Y.-D.: Estimates for the inverse elements of tridiagonal matrices. Applied Mathematics Letters 19, 590–598 (2006)

[5] Kershaw, D.: Inequalities on the elements of the inverse of a certain tridiagonal matrix. Math. Comput. 24, 155–158 (1970)

[6] Nabben, R.: Two-sided bounds on the inverse of diagonally dominant tridiagonal matrices. Linear Algebr. Appl. 287, 289–305 (1999)

[7] Yang, C.-s., Yang, S.-j.: Closure Properties of Inverse M-matrices under Hadamard Product. Journal of Anhui University (Natural Sciences) 4, 15–20 (2000)

[8] Xiu, Z., Zhang, K., Lu, Q.: Fast algorithm for Toeplitz matrix. Northwestern Polytechnical University Press (1999)

[9] Lou, X.-y., Cui, B.-t.: Exponential dissipativity of Cohen-Grossberg neural networks with mixed delays and reaction-diffusion terms 4, 619–922 (2008)

[10] Guo, X.-j., Ji, N.-h., Yao, H.-p.: The Judgement and Parallel Algorithm for Inverse M-matrixes. Journal of Beihua University 45, 97–103 (2004)

[11] Yang, Z.-y., Fu, Y.-d., Huang, T.-z.: Some Properties of InverseM-Matrices and Their Applications. Journal of UEST of China 34, 713–716 (2005)

[12] Han, Y.: The Property and Judgment of Inverse M-Matrixes. Journal of Huzhou Teachers College 30, 10–12 (2008)

[13] You, Z.: Nonsingular M-matrix. Huazhong University of Science and Technology Publishing House, Wuhan (1983)

[14] Jiang, Z.: Non singularity on scaled factor circulant matrices. Journal of Baoji College of Arts and Science (Natural Science) 23, 5–7 (2003)

[15] Li, H., Liu, X., Zhao, W.: Nonsingularity on Scaled Factor Circulant Matrices. International Journal of Algebra 2(18), 889–893 (2008)

[16] Jiang, Z.: Non singularity on r-circulant matrices. Mathematics in Practice and Theory 2, 52–58 (1995)

[17] Deng, Y.: Problem of Cyclic Matrix Inversion. Journal of Hengyang Normal University 3, 31–33 (1995)

[18] Jiang, J.: Two Simple Methods of Finding Inverse Matrix of Cyclic Matrix. Journal of Jiangxi Institute of Education(Comprehensive) 3, 5–6 (2008)

[19] Jiang, Z., Liu, S.: The Fast Algorithm for Finding the Inverse and Generalized Inverse of Permutation Factor Circulant Matrix. Numerical Mathematics A Journal of Chinese Universities 03, 227–234 (2003) (in Chinese)

[20] Cline, R.E., Plemmons, R.J., Worm, G.: Generalized inverses of certain Toeplitz matrices. Linear Algebra and Its Applications 8, 25–33 (1974)

[21] Jiang, Z., Zhou, Z.: Circulant Matrices. Chengdu Technology University Publishing Company, Chengdu (1999)

[22] Shen, G.: The Time Complexity of r-circulant Syestems. Journal Mathematical Research and Exposition 4, 595–598 (1992)

Singular Value Decomposition for k -Order Row(Column) Extended Matrix in Signal Processing

Hongkui Li

College of Science Shandong University of Technology
Shandong, 255049, People's Republic of China
lhk8068@163.com

Abstract. The row(column) extended matrices computation and the singular value decomposition of row(column) extended matrices have much important applications In this paper, motivated by the references, motivated by the references, especially [4], [5], [6], [8], we derived a quantitative correspondence of the singular values and singular vectors between the k -order row or column extended matrix A and its mother matrix, which based on the ordinary singular value decomposition, where A is nonsingular, and AA^H has distinct eigenvalues.

Keywords: row(column)extended matrix, singular value decomposition, perturbation bound.

1 Introduction

The singular value decomposition of row(column) extended matrices is necessary to understand virtually any area of mathematical science, and has been widely used in recent years. By combining hierarchy genetic algorithm with SVD(singular value decomposition), in [1], Liu Yong, Li Guangquan introduced a new RB FNN (radial basis function neural net work) training algorithm hybrid hierarchy genetic algorithm, which can greatly increases the training speed while it is still able to determine the structure and parameters of RB F from sample data, and can be used to identify and predict M-G chaos time series, and the simulation gives satisfied result. In [2], Liu Ruizhen, Tan Tieniu presented a new digital image watermarking method based on SVD(Singular Value Decomposition), and then gave some theoretical analysis about the algorithm. At last, extensive experimental results show that this method is much more robust than other methods presented before. Wang Yunhong, Tan Tieniu, Zhu Yong, in [3], proposed A face identification method based on singu lar value decomposition(SVD) and data fusion, which improves the correct verification rates from the following reasons. F irst fusion makes accurate identification results. Second, the method solves the problem of small sample size that is difficult to avoid in face recognition problem.Lastly , the LO GISTIC regression fusion method has the learning ability.So it can learn both "positive" and "negative" samples and ach ieved the correct identification rates. T he O RL face data base is used in experiment and experiment results show tha t the novel face verifica tion method is effective and possesses several desirable properties when it compared with many existing methods[3].

L. Qi (Ed.): PDCN 2010, CCIS 137, pp. 58–64, 2011.

The singular value decomposition of row(column) extended matrices, in recent years, has been studied by more and more people. In [4], The author proposed the concept of row(column) transposed matrix, analyzed the basic properties of the row(column) transposed matrix and row(column) extended matrix which leads to some new results, and gave the formula of the singular value decomposition of row(column) extended matrix, which makes the calculation easy and accurate, and saves the CPU time and memory dramatically without loss of any numerical precision. Based on the ordinary singular value decomposition, in [5], the authors derived a quantitative correspondence of the singular values and singular vectors between the row or column extended matrix (namely, the extended matrix) and its original (a k a mother matrix).

In this paper, motivated by the references, especially [4], [5], [6], [8], we derived a quantitative correspondence of the singular values and singular vectors between the k -order row or column extended matrix A and its mother matrix, which based on the ordinary singular value decomposition, where A is nonsingular, and AA^H has distinct eigenvalues.

In this paper, the matrix

$$J = \begin{pmatrix} 0 & 0 & \cdots & 0 & 1 \\ 0 & 0 & \cdots & 1 & 0 \\ \vdots & \vdots & \ddots & \vdots & \vdots \\ 0 & 1 & \cdots & & 0 \\ 1 & 0 & \cdots & 0 & 0 \end{pmatrix}$$

will denote a skew identity matrix, A^T, A^s, A^H will represent the transposed matrix, sub transposed matrix, conjugate transpose of A respectively.

Definition 1.1[8]. (k -order row extended matrix) Let $A = [a_{ij}] \in Z^{n \times n}$ be an arbitrary complex matrix, k be a given positive integer, and $P \in R^{m \times m}$ be a permutation matrix. Define matrix $R_k(P; A)$ by

$$R_k(P; A) = \begin{pmatrix} A \\ B \\ \vdots \\ B \end{pmatrix}$$

where $B = PA,$ P is permutation matrix. The matrix $R_k(P; A)$ is called the k -order row extended matrix of A , and matrix A is called the mother matrix accordingly.

Definition 1.2[8]. (k -order column extended matrix) Let $A = [a_{ij}] \in Z^{n \times n}$ be an arbitrary complex matrix, k be a given positive integer, and $P \in R^{m \times m}$ be a skew identity matrix. Define matrix $C_k(P; A)$ by

$$C_k(P;A) = [A, B, \cdots, B] \in C^{m \times kn}$$

where $B = PA$, P is permutation matrix. The matrix $C_k(P;A)$ is called the k-order column extended matrix of A, and matrix A is called the mother matrix accordingly.

2 Preliminary Notes

In this section, we present some lemmas that are important to our main results.

Lemma2.1 [5]
(1)
$$rank(R_k(P;A)) = rank(C_k(P;A)) = rank(A)$$
(2)
$$R_k(P;A)^H = C_k(P^H;A^H),$$
$$C_k(P;A)^H = R_k(P^H;A^H),$$

(3) Let $X \in C^{m \times m}, Y \in C^{n \times n}$, then
$$R_k(P;AY) = R_k(P;A)Y$$
$$C_k(P;XA) = XC_k(P;A)$$

Lemma2.2 [9]. If $A \in M_{m,n}$ has rank k, then it may be written in the form
$$A = V \Sigma W^H$$

where $V \in M_m$ and $W \in M_n$ are unitary. The matrix $\Sigma = [\sigma_{ij}] \in M_{m,n}$ has $\sigma_{ij} = 0$ for all $i \neq j$, and $\sigma_{11} \geq \sigma_{22} \geq \cdots \geq \sigma_{kk} > \sigma_{k+1,k+1} = \cdots = \sigma_{qq} = 0$, where $q = \min\{m, n\}$. The numbers $\{\sigma_{ii}\} \equiv \{\sigma_i\}$ are the nonnegative square roots of the eigenvalues of AA^H, and hence uniquely determined. The columns of V are eigenvectors of AA^H and the columns of W are eigenvectors of $A^H A$ (arranged in the same order as the same order as the corresponding eigenvalues σ_i^2). If $m \leq n$ and if AA^H has distinct eigenvalues, then V is determined up to a right diagonal factor $D = diag(e^{i\theta_1}, \cdots, e^{i\theta_n})$ with all $\theta_i \in R$; that is, if $A = V_1 \Sigma W_1^* = V_2 \Sigma W_2^*$, then $V_2 = V_1 D$. If $m < n$, then W is never uniquely determined; If $m = n = k$ and V is given, then W is uniquely determined. If $m \leq n$, the uniqueness of V and W is determined by considering A^H.

Lemma2.3 [2]. Suppose $B \in C^{m \times n}, m \geq n,$, and $B = UDV^H$ be singular value decomposition of B, where $V \in M_n$ and $W \in M_n$ are unitary, $D = \begin{pmatrix} \Sigma \\ 0 \end{pmatrix}$, $\Sigma = diag(\sigma_1, \sigma_2, \cdots, \sigma_n)$, $\sigma_1 \geq \sigma_2 \geq \cdots \geq \sigma_n \geq 0$, then there exists a singular value decompositionof the row extended matrix $A = \begin{pmatrix} B \\ J_m B \end{pmatrix} \in C^{2m \times n}$, $A = PTV^H$, where

$$T = \begin{pmatrix} D \\ 0 \end{pmatrix} = \begin{pmatrix} \sqrt{2}\Sigma \\ 0 \end{pmatrix}, \quad P = \frac{1}{\sqrt{2}} \begin{pmatrix} U & -J_m \\ J_m U & I_m \end{pmatrix}$$

3 The Main Results

In this section, we present our main results.

Theorem. Suppose $A \in M_n$, and $A = V\Sigma W^H$ be singular value decomposition of A, where $V \in M_n$ and $W \in M_n$ are unitary, $\Sigma = diag(\sigma_1, \sigma_2, \cdots, \sigma_n)$, $\sigma_1 > \sigma_2 > \cdots > \sigma_n > 0$, then the k-order row extended matrix

$$R_k(P; A) = \begin{pmatrix} A \\ B \\ \vdots \\ B \end{pmatrix} \in C^{kn \times n} \text{ exists a singular value decomposition}$$

$$R_k(P; A) = \begin{pmatrix} A \\ B \\ \vdots \\ B \end{pmatrix} = PTW^H,$$

where

$$T = \begin{pmatrix} \sqrt{k}\Sigma \\ 0 \end{pmatrix}_{kn \times n},$$

$$P = \frac{1}{\sqrt{2}} \begin{pmatrix} (A^{-1})^H W\Sigma D & -P & \cdots & -P \\ P(A^{-1})^H W\Sigma D & I_n & \cdots & 0 \\ \vdots & \vdots & \ddots & \vdots \\ P(A^{-1})^H W\Sigma D & 0 & 0 & I_n \end{pmatrix}$$

where the columns of W are eigenvectors of $A^H A$, $D = diag(e^{i\theta_1}, \cdots, e^{i\theta_n})$ with all $\theta_i \in R$.

Proof. Since $\sigma_1 > \sigma_2 > \cdots > \sigma_n > 0$, we have A is nonsingular.

By the property of AA^H, so matrix AA^H is the positive define Hermitian matrix. Now we computethe unitary diagonalization $AA^H = U \Lambda U^H$ by finding the positive eigenvalues σ_i^2 of AA^H and a corresponding set $\{u_i\}$ of normalized eigenvectors. Let

$$\tilde{U} = U = [u_1 \cdots u_n], \tilde{W} \equiv A^H \tilde{U} \Sigma^{-1},$$

Since

$$\tilde{W}\tilde{W}^H \equiv A^H \tilde{U} \Sigma^{-1}(A^H \tilde{U} \Sigma^{-1})^H = I$$

therefore $\tilde{W}$ is unitary. By the defination, we know that $A = \tilde{U} \Sigma \tilde{W}^H$ is a singular value decomposition of A.

By **Lemma2.2,** we have

$$W = \tilde{W}, V = \tilde{U} D$$

where $D = diag(e^{i\theta_1}, \cdots, e^{i\theta_n})$ with all $\theta_i \in R$, hence

$$V = (A^{-1})^H W \Sigma D$$

By the proof of **Lemma2.3,** let

$$T = \begin{pmatrix} \sqrt{k}\Sigma \\ 0 \end{pmatrix}_{kn \times n},$$

$$P = \frac{1}{\sqrt{k}} \begin{pmatrix} (A^{-1})^H W \Sigma D & -P & \cdots & -P \\ P(A^{-1})^H W \Sigma D & I_n & \cdots & 0 \\ \vdots & \vdots & \ddots & \vdots \\ P(A^{-1})^H W \Sigma D & 0 & 0 & I_n \end{pmatrix}$$

Since

$$P^H P = \left(\frac{1}{\sqrt{k}} \begin{pmatrix} (A^{-1})^H W \Sigma D & -P & \cdots & -P \\ P(A^{-1})^H W \Sigma D & I_n & \cdots & 0 \\ \vdots & \vdots & \ddots & \vdots \\ P(A^{-1})^H W \Sigma D & 0 & 0 & I_n \end{pmatrix} \right)^H \frac{1}{\sqrt{k}} \begin{pmatrix} (A^{-1})^H W \Sigma D & -P & \cdots & -P \\ P(A^{-1})^H W \Sigma D & I_n & \cdots & 0 \\ \vdots & \vdots & \ddots & \vdots \\ P(A^{-1})^H W \Sigma D & 0 & 0 & I_n \end{pmatrix} = I$$

so P is unitary, and

$$PTW^H = \frac{1}{\sqrt{k}} \begin{pmatrix} (A^{-1})^H W \Sigma D & -P & \cdots & -P \\ P(A^{-1})^H W \Sigma D & I_n & \cdots & 0 \\ \vdots & \vdots & \ddots & \vdots \\ P(A^{-1})^H W \Sigma D & 0 & 0 & I_n \end{pmatrix} \begin{pmatrix} \sqrt{k}\Sigma \\ 0 \end{pmatrix}_{kn \times n} W^H$$

$$= \begin{pmatrix} A \\ B \\ \vdots \\ B \end{pmatrix} = R_k(P; A)$$

where the columns of W are eigenvectors of $A^H A$, $D = diag(e^{i\theta_1}, \cdots, e^{i\theta_n})$ with all $\theta_i \in R$.

This completes the proof.

References

[1] Liu, Y., Li, G.: RBFNN algorithm based on hybrid hierarchy genetic algorithm and singular value decomposition. Journal of Systems Engineering 16, 486–490 (2001)

[2] Liu, R., Tan, T.: SVD Based Digital Watermarking Method. Acta Electronica Sinica 29, 168–171 (2001)

[3] Wang, Y., Tan, T., Zhu, Y.: Face Identification Based on Singular Value Decomposition and Data Fusion. Chinese J. Computers 23, 649–653 (2000)

[4] Yuan, H.: Singular Value Decomposition of Row(Column) Extended Matrix. Journal of North University of China (Natural science edition) 30, 100–104 (2009)

[5] Zou, H., Wang, D., Dai, Q., Li, Y.: Singular Value Decomposition for Extended Matrix. Chinese Science Bulletin 45, 1560–1562 (2000)

[6] Wu, Q.: Perturbation Bounds for Subunitary Polar Factors of Extended Matrix under Non-preserving Perturbation. Journal of Guangdong University of Technology 26, 86–89 (2009)

[7] Davis, K.W.: The rotation of eigenvectors by a perturbation. Numer. Anal. 7, 1–46 (1970)

[8] Zou, H., Wang, D., Dai, Q., Li, Y.: QR factorization for row or column symmetric matrix. Science in China, Ser. A 46, 83–90 (2003)

[9] Horn, R.A., Johnson, C.: Matrix Analysis. Posts & Telecom Press, Beijing (2001)

[10] Li, L., Huang, T.: Estimation for the Inverse of the Tridiagonal Matrices. Numerical Mathematics A Journal of Chinese__Universities 30, 238–244 (2009)

[11] El-Mikkawy, M.E.A.: On the inverse of a general tridiagonal matrix. Applied Mathematics and Computation 150, 669–679 (2004)

[12] Yuan, Z.: The Research on the Computing Problems and the Properties about Special Matrices. Northwestern Polytechnical University Master's Thesis (2005)

[13] Shen, G.: The Fast Algorithm for Inverting a Tridiagonal Matrix and the expression on the elements of the inverse Tridiagonal Matrix. Applied Mathematics end Mechanics 30, 238–244 (2009)

[14] Ran, R.-s., Huang, T.-z., Liu, X.-p., Gu, T.-x.: Algorithm for the Inverse of a General Tridiagonal Matrix. Applied Mathematics end Mechanics 30, 238–244 (2009)

[15] Ran, R.-s., Huang, T.-z.: Inverse of Tridiagonal Matrices. Journal of Harbin Institute of Technology 38, 815–817 (2006)

[16] Feng, J., Huang, T.-z., Liu, X.-p.: A Note on an Expression for Inverse Elements of Tridiagonal Matrix. College Mathematics 22, 103–105 (2006)

[17] Chen, J., Chen, X.: Special Matrix. Tsinghua University Press, Beijing (2001)

[18] Xiu, Z., Zhang, K., Lu, Q.: Fast algorithm for Toeplitz matrix. Northwestern Polytechnical University Press (1999)

[19] Peluso, R., Politi, T.: Some improvements for two-sided bounds on the inverse of diagonally dominant tridiagonal matrices. Linear Algebra Appl. 330, 1–14 (2001)

[20] Liu, X., Huang, T., Fu, Y.-D.: Estimates for the inverse elements of tridiagonal matrices. Applied Mathematics Letters 194, 590–598 (2006)

[21] Kershaw, D.: Inequalities on the elements of the inverse of a certain tridiagonal matrix. Math. Comput. 24, 155–158 (1970)

[22] Nabben, R.: Two-sided bounds on the inverse of diagonally dominant tridiagonal matrices. Linear Algebr. Appl. 287, 289–305 (1999)

[23] Yang, C.-s., Yang, S.-j.: Closure Properties of Inverse M-matrices under Hadamard Product. Journal of Anhui University (Natural Sciences) 4, 15–20 (2000)

[24] Lou, X.-y., Cui, B.-t.: Exponential dissipativity of Cohen-Grossberg neural networks with mixed delays and reaction-diffusion terms 4, 619–922 (2008)

[25] Guo, X.-j., Ji, N.-h., Yao, H.-p.: The Judgement and Parallel Algorithm for Inverse M-matrixes. Journal of Beihua University 45, 97–103 (2004)

Schur Decomposition for Row(Column) Extended Matrix in Signal Processing

Wenling Zhao

College of Science Shandong, University of Technology,
Shandong, 255049, People's Republic of China
zwlsdj@163.com

Abstract. The schur decomposition of row(column) extended matrices and the row(column) extended matrices computation have much important applications In this paper, motivated by the references, motivated by the references, especially [10], we derived he formula of the Schur factorization of row(column) extended matrices, which makes calculation easier and accurate.

Keywords: row(column)extended matrix, Schur decomposition, signal Processing.

1 Introduction

The schur decomposition of row(column) extended matrices is necessary to understand virtually any area of mathematical science, and has been widely used in recent years. Based on a Schur-form normal realizations, in [1], Zhu Guangxin,; Wang Kuang, Xu Hong derived an efficient structure for digital filters, which is free of self-sustained oscillations. The corresponding expression of roundoff noise gain is obtained. By two design examples, they demonstrated the superior performance of the proposed sparse structure to several well-known realizations in terms of minimizing the finite precision effects that ultimately can not be avoided in real-time applications and reducing filter implementation complexity. In [2], LIN Yu-Sheng YANG Jing-Yu presented a new face image feature extraction and recognition method-Schur Orthogonal Locality Preserving Projections (Schur-OLPP). Schur-OLPP introduces Schur decomposition in Locality Preserving Projections (LPP) to get the orthogonal vectors and extracts discriminant features. This method was tested and evaluated using the Yale face database and AR face database. Nearest neighborhood{NI} algorithm was used to construct classifiers. The experimental results show that Schur-OLPP has good performance when pose, illumination condition, face expression and time change[2].

For providing the convenient conditions for the research and design of complex high order systems, the methods often needs to reduce the model of complex systems. The order-reduction of the model of system is an important research for the design of the control system and system simulation, and is significance to the analysis, design and simulation on both theory and practice applications. Aiming at the ripe real Schur decomposition method based on system matrixes, to improve the approximation level of the reduced system , in [3], the author adopted output method, and the simulation results showed that this method can reduce the output error and was more easy and convenient for computation.

L. Qi (Ed.): PDCN 2010, CCIS 137, pp. 65–70, 2011.

By above, it is an important subject to study the theory of schur decomposition of matrix and has great significance. The research about schur decomposition of matrix is increasingly active. In [4], The author proposed the concept of row(column) transposed matrix, analyzed the basic properties of the row(column) transposed matrix and row(column) extended matrix which leads to some new results, and gave the formula of the singular value decomposition of row(column) extended matrix, which makes the calculation easy and accurate, and saves the CPU time and memory dramatically without loss of any numerical precision. Based on the ordinary singular value decomposition, in [5], the authors derived a quantitative correspondence of the singular values and singular vectors between the row or column extended matrix (namely, the extended matrix) and its original (a k a mother matrix). In[10], the author gave the concept of row(column) transposed matrix and row(column) symmetric matrix, studied the properties of the row(column) transposed matrix and row(column) symmetric matrix, and obtained the formula for the Schur factorization and normal matrix factorization of row(column) symmetric matrix.

In this paper, motivated by the references, especially [10], we derived the formula of the Schur factorization of row(column) extended matrices, which makes calculation easier and accurate.

In this paper, the matrix

$$
J = \begin{pmatrix}
0 & 0 & \cdots & 0 & 1 \\
0 & 0 & \cdots & 1 & 0 \\
\vdots & \vdots & \ddots & \vdots & \vdots \\
0 & 1 & \cdots & & 0 \\
1 & 0 & \cdots & 0 & 0
\end{pmatrix}
$$

will denote a skew identity matrix, A^T, A^s, A^H will represent the transposed matrix, sub transposed matrix, conjugate transpose of A respectively.

Definition 1.1[8]. (k-order row extended matrix) Let $A = [a_{ij}] \in Z^{n \times n}$ be an arbitrary complex matrix, k be a given positive integer, and $P \in R^{m \times m}$ be a permutation matrix. Define matrix $R_k(P; A)$ by

$$
R_k(P; A) = \begin{pmatrix}
A \\
B \\
\vdots \\
B
\end{pmatrix}
$$

where $B = PA$, P is permutation matrix. The matrix $R_k(P; A)$ is called the k-order row extended matrix of A, and matrix A is called the mother matrix accordingly.

Definition 1.2[8]. (k-order column extended matrix) Let $A = [a_{ij}] \in Z^{n \times n}$ be an arbitrary complex matrix, k be a given positive integer, and $P \in R^{m \times m}$ be a skew identity matrix. Define matrix $C_k(P; A)$ by

$$C_k(P; A) = [A, B, \cdots, B] \in C^{m \times kn}$$

where $B = PA$, P is permutation matrix. The matrix $C_k(P; A)$ is called the k-order column extended matrix of A, and matrix A is called the mother matrix accordingly.

2 Preliminary Notes

In this section, we present some lemmas that are important to our main results.

Lemma2.1 [5]

(1)

$$rank(R_k(P; A)) = rank(C_k(P; A)) = rank(A)$$

(2)

$$R_k(P; A)^H = C_k(P^H; A^H),$$

$$C_k(P; A)^H = R_k(P^H; A^H),$$

(3) Let $X \in C^{m \times m}, Y \in C^{n \times n}$, then

$$R_k(P; AY) = R_k(P; A)Y$$

$$C_k(P; XA) = XC_k(P; A)$$

Lemma2.2 [9]. (Schur) Given $A \in M_n$ with eigenvalues $\lambda_1, \cdots, \lambda_n$ in any prescribed order, there is a unitary matrix $U \in M_n$ such that

$$U^H AU = T = \begin{pmatrix} t_{11} & t_{12} & \cdots & t_{1n} \\ 0 & t_{22} & \cdots & t_{2n} \\ \vdots & \vdots & \ddots & \vdots \\ 0 & 0 & \cdots & t_{nn} \end{pmatrix}$$

is upper triangular, with diagonal entries $t_{ii} = \lambda_i$, $i = 1, 2, \cdots, n$. That is, every square matrix $A \in M_n$ is unitarily equivalent to a triangular matrix whose diagonal entries are the eigenvalent of $A \in M_n$ in a prescribed order. Furthermore, if $A \in M_n(R)$ and if all the eigenvalues of $A \in M_n$ are real, then $U \in M_n$ may be chosen tobe real and orthogonal.

Lemma2.3 [2]. Suppose $B \in C^{m \times n}, m \geq n,$, and $B = UDV^H$ be singular value decomposition of B, where $V \in M_n$ and $W \in M_n$ are unitary, $D = \begin{pmatrix} \Sigma \\ 0 \end{pmatrix}$, $\Sigma = diag(\sigma_1, \sigma_2, \cdots, \sigma_n)$, $\sigma_1 \geq \sigma_2 \geq \cdots \geq \sigma_n \geq 0$, then there exists a singular value decompositionof the row extended matrix $A = \begin{pmatrix} B \\ J_m B \end{pmatrix} \in C^{2m \times n}$,

$A = PTV^H$, where

$$T = \begin{pmatrix} D \\ 0 \end{pmatrix} = \begin{pmatrix} \sqrt{2}\Sigma \\ 0 \end{pmatrix}, \quad P = \frac{1}{\sqrt{2}} \begin{pmatrix} U & -J_m \\ J_m U & I_m \end{pmatrix}$$

3 The Main Results

In this section, we present our main results.

Theorem. Suppose $A \in M_n$, and $A = U^H TU$ be the Schur decomposition of A,

where $U \in M_n$ is unitary, $T = \begin{pmatrix} t_{11} & t_{12} & \cdots & t_{1n} \\ 0 & t_{22} & \cdots & t_{2n} \\ \vdots & \vdots & \ddots & \vdots \\ 0 & 0 & \cdots & t_{nn} \end{pmatrix}$ is upper triangular, with

diagonal entries $t_{ii} = \lambda_i$, $i = 1, 2, \cdots, n$., then the 2-order row extended matrix $R_2(P; A) = \in C^{2n \times n}$ exists a decomposition

$$R_2(P; A) = QLU^H,$$

where

$$L = \begin{pmatrix} \sqrt{2}T \\ 0 \end{pmatrix}_{2n \times n},$$

$$Q = \frac{1}{\sqrt{2}} \begin{pmatrix} U & U \\ PU & -PU \end{pmatrix}$$

is unitary.

Proof. The proof is simulaly to [10].

Firstly,

$$QLU^H = \frac{1}{\sqrt{2}} \begin{pmatrix} U & U \\ PU & -PU \end{pmatrix} \begin{pmatrix} \sqrt{2}T \\ 0 \end{pmatrix}_{2n \times n} U^H$$

$$= \frac{1}{\sqrt{2}} \begin{pmatrix} \sqrt{2}UT \\ \sqrt{2}PUT \end{pmatrix}_{2n \times n} U^H$$

$$= \begin{pmatrix} UTU^H \\ PUTU^H \end{pmatrix}_{2n \times n} = R_2(P;A)$$

At last, we prove Q is unitary.

$$Q^H Q = \left(\frac{1}{\sqrt{2}} \begin{pmatrix} U & U \\ PU & -PU \end{pmatrix} \right)^H \frac{1}{\sqrt{2}} \begin{pmatrix} U & U \\ PU & -PU \end{pmatrix}$$

$$= \frac{1}{\sqrt{2}} \begin{pmatrix} U^H & U^H P^H \\ U^H & -U^H P^H \end{pmatrix} \frac{1}{\sqrt{2}} \begin{pmatrix} U & U \\ PU & -PU \end{pmatrix}$$

$$= \frac{1}{2} \begin{pmatrix} 2I_n & 0 \\ 0 & 2I_n \end{pmatrix} = I_{2n}$$

This completes the proof.

References

[1] Zhu, G., Wang, K., Xu, H.: A New Method of Fisher Discriminant Analysis with Schur Decomposition. Journal of Circuits and Systems 15, 1–5 (2010)

[2] Lin, Y.-S., Yang, J.-Y.: A New Method of Fisher Discriminant Analysis with Schur Decomposition. Computer Science 23, 702–705 (2007)

[3] Meng, Q.: Ordered real Schur decomposition method of model reduction based on system matrixes. Information Technology 6, 49–52 (2006)

[4] Yuan, H.: Singular Value Decomposition of Row(Column) Extended Matrix. Journal of North University of China (Natural science edition) 30, 100–104 (2009)

[5] Zou, H., Wang, D., Dai, Q., Li, Y.: Singular Value Decomposition for Extended Matrix. Chinese Science Bulletin 45, 1560–1562 (2000)

[6] Wu, Q.: Perturbation Bounds for Subunitary Polar Factors of Extended Matrix under Non-preserving Perturbation. Journal of Guangdong University of Technology 26, 86–89 (2009)

[7] Davis, K.W.: The rotation of eigenvectors by a perturbation. Numer. Anal. 7, 1–46 (1970)

[8] Zou, H., Wang, D., Dai, Q., Li, Y.: QR factorization for row or column symmetric matrix. Science in China, Ser. A 46, 83–90 (2003)

[9] Horn, R.A., Johnson, C.: Matrix Analysis. Posts & Telecom Press, Beijing (2001)

[10] Yuan, H.: Schur factorization and normal matrices factorization of row(column)symmetric matrices. Journal of Shandong University(Natural Science) 42, 1–4 (2007)

[11] Li, L., Huang, T.: Estimation for the Inverse of the Tridiagonal Matrices. Numerical Mathematics A Journal of Chines__Universities 30, 238–244 (2009)

[12] El-Mikkawy, M.E.A.: On the inverse of a general tridiagonal matrix. Applied Mathematics and Computation 150, 669–679 (2004)

[13] Yuan, Z.: The Research on the Computing Problems and the Properties about Special Matrices, Northwestern Polytechnical University Master's Thesis (2005)

[14] Shen, G.: The Fast Algorithm for Inverting a Tridiagonal Matrix and the expression on the elements of the inverse Tridiagonal Matrix. Applied Mathematics and Mechanics 30, 238–244 (2009)

[15] Ran, R.-s., Huang, T.-z., Liu, X.-p., Gu, T.-x.: Algorithm for the Inverse of a General Tridiagonal Matrix. Applied Mathematics and Mechanics 30, 238–244 (2009)

[16] Ran, R.-s., Huang, T.-z.: Inverse of Tridiagonal Matrices. Journal of Harbin Institute of Technology 38, 815–817 (2006)

[17] Feng, J., Huang, T.-z., Liu, X.-p.: A Note on an Expression for Inverse Elements of Tridiagonal Matrix. College Mathematics 22, 103–105 (2006)

[18] Chen, J., Chen, X.: Special Matrix. Tsinghua University Press, Beijing (2001)

[19] Xiu, Z., Zhang, K., Lu, Q.: Fast algorithm for Toeplitz matrix. Northwestern Polytechnical University Press (1999)

[20] Peluso, R., Politi, T.: Some improvements for two-sided bounds on the inverse of diagonally dominant tridiagonal matrices. Linear Algebra Appl. 330, 1–14 (2001)

[21] Liu, X., Huang, T., Fu, Y.-D.: Estimates for the inverse elements of tridiagonal matrices. Applied Mathematics Letters 194, 590–598 (2006)

[22] Kershaw, D.: Inequalities on the elements of the inverse of a certain tridiagonal matrix. Math. Comput. 24, 155–158 (1970)

[23] Nabben, R.: Two-sided bounds on the inverse of diagonally dominant tridiagonal matrices. Linear Algebr. Appl. 287, 289–305 (1999)

[24] Yang, C.-s., Yang, S.-j.: Closure Properties of Inverse M-matrices under Hadamard Product. Journal of Anhui University (Natural Sciences) 4, 15–20 (2000)

[25] Lou, X.-y., Cui, B.-t.: Exponential dissipativity of Cohen-Grossberg neural networks with mixed delays and reaction-diffusion terms 4, 619–922 (2008)

[26] Guo, X.-j., Ji, N.-h., Yao, H.-p.: The Judgement and Parallel Algorithm for Inverse M-matrixes. Journal of Beihua University 45, 97–103 (2004)

Prolog-Based Formal Reasoning for Security Protocols

Rongrong Jiang[1,2], Chuanbin Wang[2], Jiejie Xu[2], and Jiangfen Yu[1]

[1] College of Inforamtion and Engineering, Zhejiang Radio & Television University,
Hangzhou, 310030, China
[2] Zhejiang Key Laboratory of Inforamtion Security, Hangzhou, 310012, China

Abstract. This paper introduces a security reachability analysis model based on the strand space theory and the constraint elimination method. A prolog-based automatic reasoning scheme is then proposed. At last, the reasoning implementation utilizing the Java interface of XSB (a prolog interpreter) is described.

Keywords: Formal method, Security protocols, Prolog, Automatic reasoning.

1 Introduction

Since the BAN logic[1]appeared ,the formal analysis techniques for security protocols have been greatly concerned, such as logic reasoning, state machine model, algebraic system, etc.[2]. It is accepted the strand space model [3] is a novel and promising method, which combines theorem and the track of protocols. The security of protocol can be analyzed itself through the reachability[4]. It is not considered secure if the security protocol can reach a certain state of insecurity from the initial state. In this paper, the parties of public information of the protocol will be used to initialize the strand space to build the model of congregate restriction of protocols [5]. It can then use the prolog to realize the automatic reasoning of the process for constraint reduction. Thinks to that the automation analysis tool of security protocols is a hard but hot research topic [6], the prolog interpreter XSB for Java is finally used to realize the prototype for formal reasoning on security protocols.

2 The Reachability of Strand Space Method

2.1 Message Items

Denote the information exchanged by all principals of security protocols as the message item sets A. Message item A can be divided into specific message items (such as principal ID, random number, etc.) and key message items (including symmetric keys, asymmetric keys, etc.). Message item sets A also can be divided into explicit information item sets T and key messages item sets K.

We first give the following symbols items which will be following employed.

(1) ε the attacker.
(2) $[t_1, t_2]$ news couple.

L. Qi (Ed.): PDCN 2010, CCIS 137, pp. 71–77, 2011.
© Springer-Verlag Berlin Heidelberg 2011

(3) $pk(P)$ the public key of principal P (Assuming an attacker cannot access to P's private key, attacker ε can only decrypt the information encrypted by $pk(\varepsilon)$.

(4) $h(t)$ The hash value of message t.

(5) $[t]_k^{\leftrightarrow}$ The message t encrypted by the symmetric key k.

(6) $sig_k(t)$ The message t signed by the private key k.

2.2 Strand Space Definitions

There are two type of messages in protocol implementations, message sent and message received. Therefore, we can define the messages with symbols for binary groups $< s, a >$ where $a \in A, s = +$ means sending messages, $s = -$ means receiving messages. So $< s, a >$ is generally abbreviated as $+a$ or $-a$.

String is a sequence of events that a principal may be participated. For Legitimate principals, each string is a series of receiving and sending information on behalf of behaviors in the implement progress of specific protocols, as well as all message item values. The attacker string is a message sequence that the attacker may to send and receive. The strand space is defined as an aggregation Σ that contains a variety of legitimate main string and attacker strings with a track map denoted as

$$tr : \Sigma \rightarrow (\pm A)^* .$$

(1) Nodes $n =< s, i >$, which $s \in \Sigma, 1 \leq i \leq lengthen(s) . n \in s$ means n belongs to string s. Each node belongs to the only string and N means the node set.

(2) If $n =< s, i > \in N$ that $index(n) = i, term(n) = (tr(s))i, strand(n) = s$.

(3) If $n_1, n_2 \in N$,that $n_1 \rightarrow n_2$,so $term(n_1) = +a$ and $term(n_2) = -a$,means n_1 sends messages to n_2 . It is an expression of the sequence between different strings.

(4) If $n_1, n_2 \in N$,that $n_1 \Rightarrow n_2$,so $term(n_1) = +a$ and $term(n_2) = -a$,means n_1 and n_2 appear in the same string, and to satisfy $index(n_1) = index(n_2) - 1$ that means n_1 is the direct precessor of n_2 .

(5) No symbol item t appeared at $n \in N$ only when $t \subset term(n)$.

(6) Define I is no symbol item node $n \in N$ is the entry point for I ,only when $term(n) = +t$,$t \in I$,and $n' \Rightarrow +n, term(n') \not\subset I$.

(7) No symbol item t comes from $n \in N$ only when the sign of $term(n)$ is positive, $t \subset term(n)$ and to any processor of node of n, $m, t \notin term(m)$.

2.3 Parameter Strand and Reachability

Parameter string is just a specific type of the string mentioned above. It is the event sequence of principals, usually includes message items be sent and received. The difference to others is that it contains a number of variables, and different variables can discriminate different strings. For example, for the well-known NSL[7] protocol the parameters string of sponsors of protocols can be described as follows.

$$Init(A, B, N_A, N_B) = +[A, N_A]^{\rightarrow}_{pk(B)} - [N_A, N_B, B]^{\rightarrow}_{pk(A)} + [N_B]^{\rightarrow}_{pk(B)}$$

The way of the parameter string of receivers $\operatorname{Re} sp(A, B, N_A, N_B)$ is not the same, the diffidence is exchange $+$ and $-$ exchange.

$[x]^{\rightarrow}_{pk(A)}$ means use the public key of parameter(Initiator) to encrypt message x.

$+$ and $-$ mean to send and receive the messages, combining both is with a node, for example $+[N_B]^{\rightarrow}_{pk(B)}$, messages item is usually expressed by the capital letters, for example N_B.

We will use mitigation measures to analysis parameters string set. Just call the parameter string is semi-bundle. Nodes of each string in the sequence implied the change of status among principals, that $\{Init(A, B, N_A, N_B), \operatorname{Re} sp(A', B', N'_A, N'_B)\}$ is a semi-bundle, each string in semi-bundle need not to be completed, it maybe a substring of string parameters of principals.

If a semi-bundle is complete, it shows that the bundle state can be achieve from the initial state, that is, the semi-bundle is attainability. Semi-bundle complete or not can be used to describe the attack, if the attacker can, through appropriate initialization, through some algorithm to reach a safe state (usually the confidential information of protocol leakage) show that protocol unsafe. Through this we can determine the security of protocols through the accessibility.

3 Constraint Reduction Method

3.1 Constraint Set

Constraint set use $m : T$ to express, m means a message item, T means a message set, T on behalf of the message set that the attacker know, the attacker use the information of T to compose m. The node with "$+$" can be added to the final set of message items T, and the node with "$-$" can be used to bound a new construct set $m : T$.

The initial message set A contains the initial information, assumpt that the attacker will get the initial information, eg : the ID of A,B (a, b), the ID of attacker and the public key （$\varepsilon, pk(\varepsilon)$） and so on. So T can be as $\{a, b, pk(a), pk(b), \varepsilon, pk(\varepsilon)\}$ and so on. As NSL protocol, constraint set can be expressed as follows:

$$[A, B] : T_0 = \{a, b, \varepsilon, pk(\varepsilon)\}$$

$$[a, N_A]_{pk(b)}^{\rightarrow} : T_1 = T_0 \cup \{[A, na]_{pk(B)}^{\rightarrow}\}$$

$$[na, N_B, B]_{pk(A)}^{\rightarrow} : T_2 = T_1 \cup \{[N_A, nb, b]_{pk(a)}^{\rightarrow}\}$$

$$nb : T_3 = T_2 \cup \{[N_B]_{pk(B)}^{\rightarrow}\}$$

3.2 Constraint Reduction

Based on the reduction rules, each constraint set will be decomposed or replaced partly in the process of reduction , it may replaced by other constants , or or to replace a whole, or broken down into more sub- constraint set. If the left of constraint set is a variable, so called the constraint set is a simple constraint set, or Non-abatement constraint set.

A constraint set may have more than one mitigation measures, it can use the tree structure (reduction tree) to analysis. We can create a root node C_0 in the initial constraint set in the process of abatement constraints. C_0 is a simple constraint set ,it may be a way to attack the protocol too.

A reduction tree is set by the constraint as nodes, reduction rules as sides to build. Tree root node is the initial constraint set C , including C_0. Specific abatement process P as follows.

(1) $C^* = m : T$ is a restriction in constraint set , and m is not a variable . If C^* cann't be found , that it is able to meet , or use reduction rules to C^*, enumerate of all possible constraint.
(2)   Use reduction rules r on C, if match, set $<C; \sigma'> := r(C, \sigma)$, create a new node C', add the node in the recursive stack.
(3)   Repeat steps (1) and (2). $C; \sigma$ means the sate in the process of reduction . C is the current constraint set, σ means the replace some variables in the constraint set.

3.3 Reduction Rules and Examples

To the cryptographic assumptions of security protocols, following reduction rules are proposed.

$$\frac{C_<, m : T \ , \ C_>, \sigma}{\tau C_< , \tau C_> , \tau \cup \sigma} \tag{1}$$

$$where \ \tau = mgu(m, t), t \in T;$$

$$\frac{C_<, [m_1, m_2] : T, C_>, \sigma}{C_<, m_1 : T, m_2 : T, C_>, \sigma} \tag{2}$$

$$\frac{C_<\,h(m):T,C_>,\sigma}{C_<\,m:T,C_>,\sigma} \tag{3}$$

$$\frac{C_<\,[m]_k^\rightarrow:T,C_>,\sigma}{C_<\,k:T,m:T,C_>,\sigma} \tag{4}$$

$$\frac{C_<\,[m]_k^\leftrightarrow:T,C_>,\sigma}{C_<\,k:T,m:T,C_>,\sigma} \tag{5}$$

$$\frac{C_<\,sig_{pk(\varepsilon)}(m):T,C_>,\sigma}{C_<\,m:T,C_>,\sigma} \tag{6}$$

$$\frac{C_<\,m:[t_1,t_2]\cup T,C_>,\sigma}{C_<\,m:t_1\cup t_2\cup T,C_>,\sigma} \tag{7}$$

$$\frac{C_<\,m:[t]_{pk(\varepsilon)}^\rightarrow\cup T,C_>,\sigma}{C_<\,m:t\cup T,C_>,\sigma} \tag{8}$$

$$\frac{C_<\,m:[t]_k^\rightarrow\cup T,C_>,\sigma}{\tau C_<\,\tau m:\tau[t]_k^\rightarrow\cup\tau T,\tau C_>,\tau\cup\sigma} \tag{9}$$

$$where\ \tau=mgu(k,pk(\varepsilon)),k\neq pk(\varepsilon)$$

The examples illustrate how to use abatement rules to analysis the security of NSL protocol. First, give a description of NSL.

a. $A\rightarrow B:\{N_A,A\}_{pk(B)}^\rightarrow$

b. $B\rightarrow A:\{B,N_A,N_B\}_{pk(A)}^\rightarrow$

c. $A\rightarrow B:\{N_B\}_{pk(B)}^\rightarrow$

We consider the parameter string that exchanged by the receiver b and sponsor A (lower case on behalf of constant capital on behalf of variables). The final step of protocol have been omitted, more the strings are contained in the semi-string for analysis. We add a secret information receive string $-nb$ to the final of the string, to test whether nb has been leaked in the process.Interactive constraint set as follow.

$$[a,N_A]_{pk(b)}^\rightarrow:T_0=\{a,b,\varepsilon,pk(a),pk(b)\}$$

$$[B,N_B]_{pk(A)}^\rightarrow:T_1=T_0\cup\{[N_A,[nb,b]]_{pk(a)}^\rightarrow\}$$

$$nb:T_1\cup\{[N_B,[na,A]]_{pk(B)}^\rightarrow\}$$

Based on Rule (4) and message a we can get:

1.1 $pk(b):T_0$

1.2 $[a,N_A]:T_0$

Based on Rule (1) on (1.1) and Rule (2) on (1.2) we can get:

1.2.1 $a : T_0$

1.2.2 $N_A : T_0$

Based on Rule (4) on (1.2.1) and message b we can get:

$$B \rightarrow N_A, N_B \rightarrow [nb, b], A \rightarrow a .$$

Based on Rule (9) and message c we can get:

$$N_A \rightarrow \varepsilon$$

It finally shows that nb is not safe, and the protocol is at security risk.

4 Reasoning Using Prolog

Prolog has been widely used in the natural language understanding, machine theorem proving, and expert systems, the paper will use Prolog to realize that automatic reasoning and analysis the security protocols.

Strand space express the sequence of events that the parties of protocol may participate in. All sequence of events of the parties of protocol can be expressed through prolog, such as NSPK protocol , the sequence of events of A in the protocol are expressed as follow:

$$Init(A, B, N_A, N_B) = +[A, N_A]_{pk(B)}^{\rightarrow} - [N_A, N_B, B]_{pk(A)}^{\rightarrow} + [N_B]_{pk(B)}^{\rightarrow}$$

Use Prolog to express as follow:

```
strand(roleA,A,B,Na,Nb,[
  recv([A,B]),
  send([A,Na]*pk(B)),
  recv([Na,Nb]*pk(A)),
  send(Nb*pk(B))
]).
```

Abatement rules used in analysis of the protocol can be expressed through prolog. As prolog can automatic recursion and remount, there is no need to consider the process of running processes. Just to consider the logical relationship. XSB system will be used in this article, XSB is a logic language reasoning system for business research ,it support the standard syntax of prolog.

XSB can be used to realize the abatement rules, for example:

reduct ([A,B],T,[[B,T],[A,T]]) :- !. means pair rules, analyze [A,B]->[B,T]U[A,T]: reduct(M/pk(e),T,[[M,T]]) :- !.means Rule (4), as it is the ideograph of public key e,M can be added into C;

```
reduct(M,T,[]) :-
member(A,T),
hunify(M,A).
```

means Rule (1) , use Hunify predication to add M into C.

Other rules may also be realized in similar ways, we will not repeat here.

5   Conclusion

The formal method based on strand space is a new way to analyze security protocols. It is more convenient, efficient, and easier to be extended than that of traditional BAN logics. For measures to digest restriction, adding constraint digest rules can enhance the analytical capacity of the model protocol. Future work will focus on the strategy of achievement and the process of implementation, as well as to improve the power of automatic analysis supported by prolog-based tools.

Acknowledgments. This work is partially supported by the 2009 Zhejiang Provincial Education Research Project under grant No.Y200909152.

References

1. Burrows, M., Abadi, M., Needham, R.: A logic of authentication. Proceedings of the Royal Society of London A 426, 233–271 (1989)
2. Qin, S.: Twenty years development of security protocols research. Journal of Software 14(10), 2036–2044 (2003)
3. Fábrega, F., Herzog, J., Guttman, J.: Strand spaces: Proving security protocols correct. Journal of Computer Security 7(2,3), 191–230 (1999)
4. Jonathan, M., Shmatikov, V.: Constraint solving for bounded-process cryptographic protocol analysis. In: 8th ACM Conference on Computer and Communications Security, pp. 166–175. ACM Press, Philadelphia (2001)
5. Amadio, R.M., Vincent, V., et al.: On the symbolic reduction of processes with cryptographic functions. Theory of Computer Science 290(1), 695–740 (2003)
6. Chen, T., Cai, J.: Research on visual analysis and design of security protocols. Journal of Communication and Computer 2(12), 27–31 (2005)
7. Amadio, R.M., Lugiez, D.: On the reachability problem in cryptographic protocols. In: Proceedings of the 11th International Conference, August 2000. Springer, Heidelberg (2000)
8. Lowe, G.: Breaking and Fixing the Needham-Sc-hroeder Public-Key Protocol Using FDR. In: Proceedings of the Second International Workshop, March 1996. Springer, Heidelberg (1996)
9. Song, D.X.: A New Efficient Automatic Checker for Security Protocol Analysis. In: IEEE Computer Security Foundations Workshop 1999. IEEE Computer Society, Los Alamitos (1999)

Development of SOPC-Based Wireless Sensor Nodes in Farmland

Ken Cai[1,2,*] and Xiaoying Liang[3]

[1] School of Bioscience and Bioengineering,
South China University of Technology, Guangzhou 510641, China
[2] Information College,
Zhongkai University of Agriculture and Engineering, Guangzhou 510225, China
[3] Guangdong Women's Polytechnic College, Guangzhou 511450, China
{caiken218,minnielxy}@gmail.com

Abstract. Wireless Sensor Network (WSN) is a product that unifies sensor technology, embedded computing technology, distributed information technology and wireless communication technology. At present it already is foreseen that it would have widespread application domain and high value. The main research contents of this paper include: the design of wireless sensor nodes, the method of hardware-software co-design, the reuse and design of embedded IP cores, the date acquisition, and the communication network and so on. Firstly, the performance requirement and development trend of wireless multimedia sensor nodes are analyzed. For the application of farmland information monitoring system, one wireless sensor node based on the SOPC is proposed, which designed with the Nios II processor, wireless communication chip CC2430 and some sensors. The hardware circuit diagram of each main module is given. Secondly, some IP cores in the bottom of WSN are designed and implemented, which are the important parts of In-Node Processing and In-Node Communicating. Finally, the software framework of wireless sensor nodes based on SOPC is analyzed, and the main work flow diagram of the system is provided in the paper.

Keywords: Sensor, Wireless transmission, Farmland, SOPC, FPGA.

1 Introduction

With the rapid developing of electronics, communication and embedded system technologies, sensor networks are applied to various fields ranging from special application fields such as environmental pollution, landscape flooding alarm, soil moisture monitoring, and microclimate and solar radiation mapping to daily application fields such as fire monitoring and pollution monitoring [1], [2].They are playing more and more important roles in collaborative real-time monitoring. The information from environment are collected and transferred to user terminals after some necessary processing. The new generation sensor networks are constructed by three parts (a radio transceiver, a power system and a micro controller). Radio transceiver is

* This research was supported by Guangdong Provincial Science and Technology Planning Project of China under grant 2010B020315028.

L. Qi (Ed.): PDCN 2010, CCIS 137, pp. 78–84, 2011.
© Springer-Verlag Berlin Heidelberg 2011

responsible for the communication. The task of the micro controller is to control the sensors and process the data. All the powers needed for transceiver and micro controller are coming from power system such as battery and solar power. Comparing with the traditional wire mode, the new wireless sensor networks overcome much more disadvantages, such as complex wiring, high power, poor reliability, poor real-time capability, difficult maintenance and so on[3],[4],[5].

On the other hand, with the rapid development of semiconductor technology, the single chip capacity of FPGA (Field Programmable Gate Array) increases greatly whereas its power consumption decreases tremendously, which has become a hot technology and it has been widely used in practice [6]. IP designs can be developed and downloaded into FPGA to work with an embedded processor, which called system-on-a-programmable-chip (SOPC) technology [7]. Altera's SOPC builder development tool dramatically simplifies the task of creating high-performance SOPC designs by accelerating system definition and integration. Using SOPC Builder, system designers can define and implement a complete system, including generating all the interconnect logic required to connect the system components in the manner, within one tool and in a fraction of the time of traditional system-on-a-chip (SoC) design. The use of this design methodology offers significant benefit to the design team through composing bus based systems from common system components placed inside or outside the FPGA and hence, increased focus on system development and verification [8]. Furthermore, due to low processing power, slow operation speed and the limited available I/O port of the MCU, choosing the high performance FPGA chip can be a good solution, and also can shorten the product development cycles significantly and improve the development efficiency.

In this paper, we present the design of a novel wireless sensor node based on a low-cost, low-power FPGA (Altera EP2C35 FPGA). This node features dynamic reconfiguration capabilities, high adaptivity, small size, powerful data processing ability and high rate wireless communication ability. This new architecture offers significant flexibility to deal with the trade-offs between processing and communication. In addition, in our proposed paradigm, a large number of sensor nodes are densely deployed in farmland. The measured data (e.g., temperature, relative humidity) is collected by sensor nodes and sent to their respective cluster nodes that collaboratively process the data. This makes the wireless sensor node applicable to outdoor environment and any other monitoring of the dynamic system state.

The remaining paper is organized as follows: In the section 2, we discuss our proposed system architecture. In section 3, we present design architecture of a wireless sensor node, containing temperature sensors design, humidity sensors design, the wireless communication module design, and CMOS image sensor design, etc. In Section 4, we draw the conclusion along with an indication of future work.

2 System Architecture Design

The hardware structure of SOPC-based wireless sensor nodes comprises the Cyclone development board, sensor signal modulation circuit, CMOS image sensor, etc. The core control unit consists of a Cyclone EP2C35 FPGA, DDR SDRAM, flash memory, UART interface, USB-Blaster download interface, clock, configuration circuit, power, etc. Figure 1 shows the system hardware block diagram.

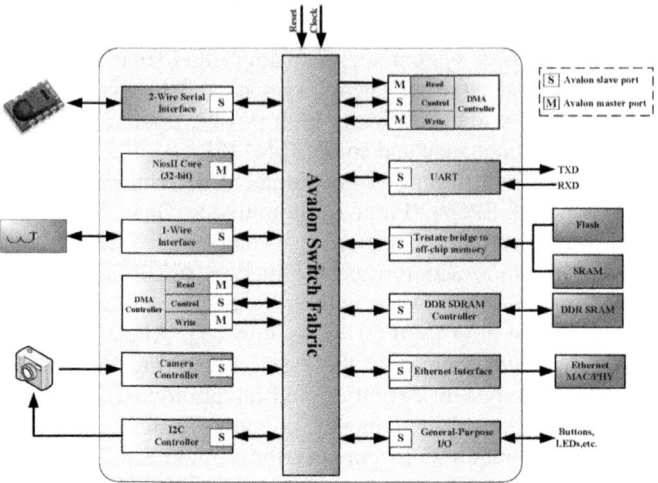

Fig. 1. System Hardware Block Diagram

3 Implementation

3.1 Temperature Sensors Design

The temperature sensors used in this design are high precision digital sensors DS18B20 in 1-Wire series of Dallas Company, which has an operating temperature

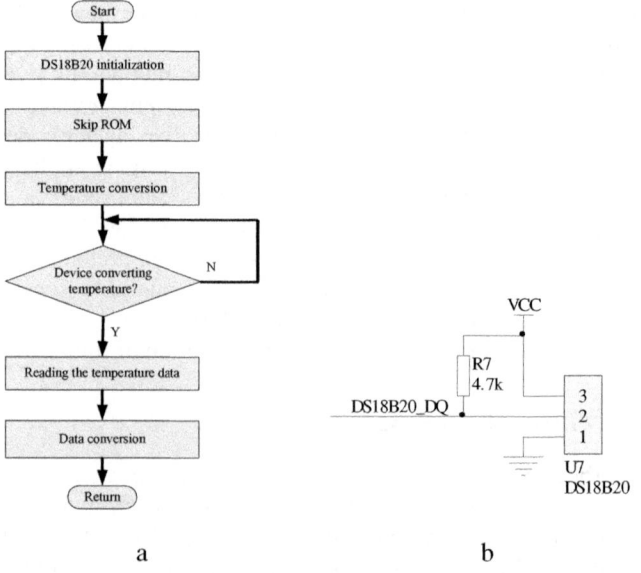

Fig. 2. (a) Temperature acquisition flow chart. (b) Schematic circuit diagram of DS18B20.

range of -55°C to +125°C and is accurate to ±0.5°C over the range of -10°C to +85°C. The DS18B20 digital thermometer provides 9-bit to 12-bit Celsius temperature measurements and has an alarm function with nonvolatile user-programmable upper and lower trigger points. The DS18B20 communicates over a 1-Wire bus. Different from most of the current standard serial data communication means (such as SPI, I2C, etc.), 1-Wire bus uses single signal lines to transmit not only the clock but also data. This system is to use DS18B20 to achieve farmland ambient temperature measurement. Figure 2 shows temperature acquisition flow chart and circuit of DS18B20.

3.2 Humidity Sensors Design

The humidity sensor uses SHT11 which is Sensirion's family of surface mountable relative humidity and temperature sensors. It has many characteristics, such as integrating sensor elements plus signal processing on a tiny foot print, providing a fully calibrated digital output, programmable regulation of measurement resolution (8/12/14 bit data), etc. It provides 2-wire serial interface and internal voltage regulation to allow for easy and fast system integration. The tiny size and low power consumption makes SHT11 the ultimate choice for even the most demanding applications. Figure 3 shows temperature acquisition flow chart and circuit of SHT11.

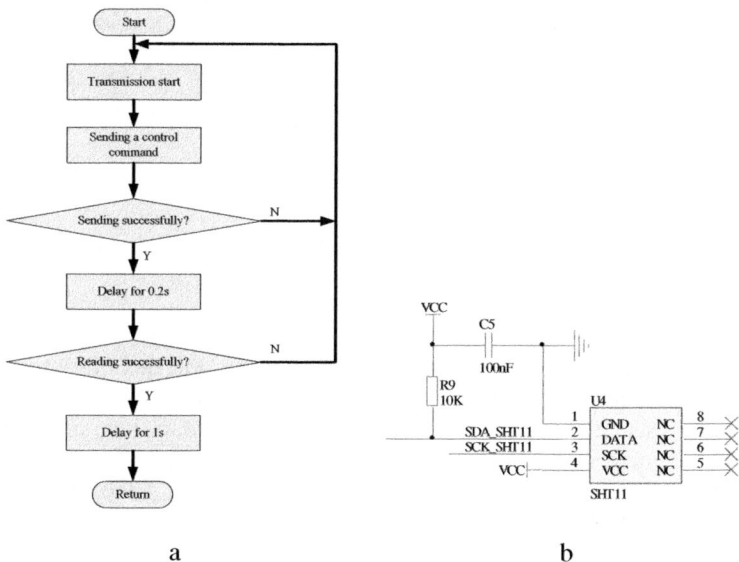

a   b

Fig. 3. (a) Humidity acquisition flow chart. (b) Schematic circuit diagram of SHT11.

3.3 The Wireless Communication Module Design

CC2430 is a true resolution to System-on-Chip (SoC), which can improve performance and meet the requirements of IEEE 802.15.4 and ZigBee applications on low costs and low power consumption. The CC2430 comes in three different flash versions: CC2430F32/64/128(32/64/128 KB flash). It enables ZigBee nodes to be built with very low total bill-of-material costs, and combines the excellent performance of the leading CC2420 RF transceiver with an industrial-grade compact and efficient 8051 MCU. The enhanced 8051 MCU has 128KB programmable flash memory, 8KB RAM, and many other powerful features. Using the industry leading ZigBee protocol stack (Z-Stack) from Texas Instruments, the CC2430 provides the market's most competitive ZigBee solution. The CC2430 is highly suited for those applications requiring a very long battery life. Figure 4 shows ZigBee sensor node flow chart and circuit of CC2430.

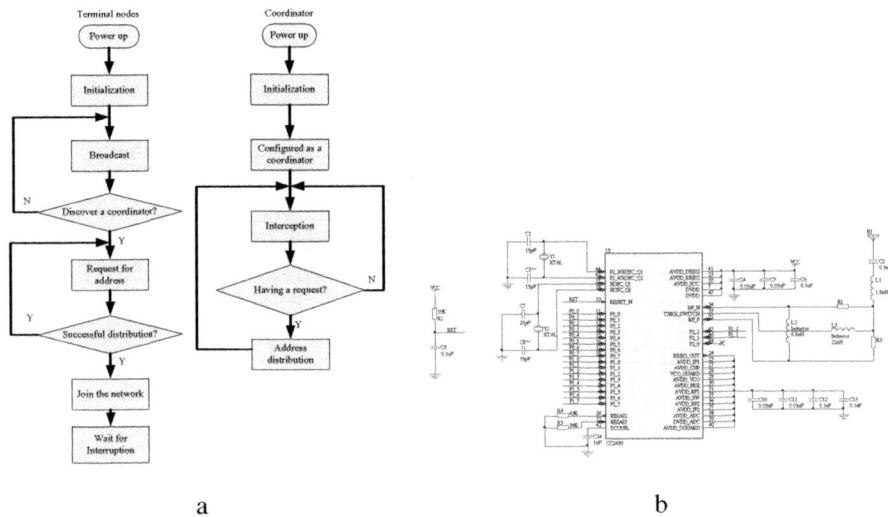

a   b

Fig. 4. (a) ZigBee sensor node flow chart. (b) Schematic circuit diagram of CC2430.

3.4   CMOS Image Sensor Design

Implementing a camera controller in an FPGA provides the flexibility to incorporate additional camera module features quickly and easily as they become available. This controller consists of three modules, including a video data bus and some control signals. The camera controller allows sending the acquired video data towards the FIFO module with 32 Bits word. Figure 5 shows structure of the camera control IP core and circuit of CMOS camera.

3.5   System Architecture Implementation

We used Altera's SOPC Builder to build the system. The system is configured with a GUI (Figure 6) and different SOPC Builder components (DDR SDRAM controller, Nios II processor, UART, ect.) are instantiated around the Avalon memory-mapped (Avalon-MM) bus. SOPC Builder provides files to the Quartus II software for the FPGA configuration elaboration. It also provides files to the Nios II software development tools to build a specific board support package (BSP) library.

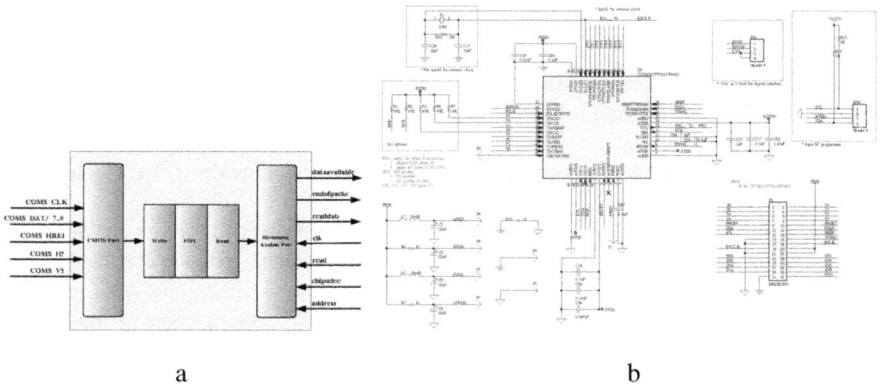

a   b

Fig. 5. (a) Structure of the camera control IP core. (b) Schematic circuit diagram of CMOS camera.

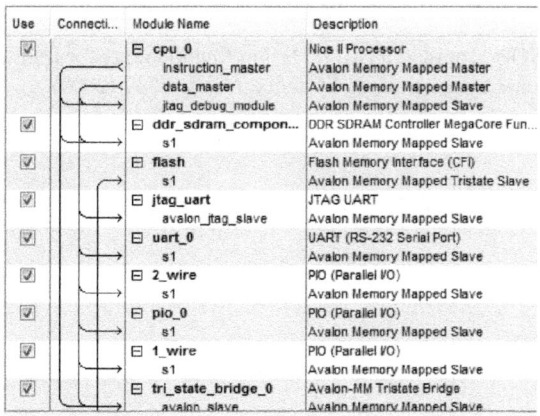

Fig. 6. Nios II processor and hardware modules in SOPC Builder

4   Conclusion and Future Works

Using the SOPC technology, we have created a novel design and implementation method of the wireless sensor nodes for farmland information management system. It consists of the Nios II soft-core processor, the temperature sensor, the relative humidity sensor, the CMOS image sensor and the RF module so on. Comparing with other traditional design, our system can realize the rapid expansion and on-line upgrade capability, which greatly reduces the time and the cost of product update. In the future, we will further focus on the work on improving the system speed, transfer efficiency, image compression and the total energy spent in transmission and processing.

References

1. Haenselman, T.: Sensornetworks, GFDL (2006)
2. Cook, D., Das, S.: Smart Environments: Technology, Protocols, and Applications. Wiley, Chichester (2004)
3. Culler, D., Estrin, D., Srivastava, M.: Overview of sensor networks. IEEE Computer 37(8), 41–49 (2004)
4. Feng, J., Koushanfar, F., Potkonjak, M.: System-architectures for sensor networks issues, alternatives, and directions. In: IEEE International Conference on Computer Design (ICCD) (2002)
5. Raja, K., Daskalopoulos, I., Diall, H., Hailes, S., Torfs, T.: Sensor cubes: a modular, ultra-compact, power-aware platform for sensor networks. In: International Conference on Information Processing in Sensor Networks (IPSN SPOTS) (2006)
6. Shang, L., Kaviani, A.S., Bathala, K.: Dynamic Power Consumption in Virtex-II FPGA Family. In: Proceedings of the 2002 ACM/SIGDA 10th International Symposium on Field-Programmable Gate Arrays, pp. 157–164. ACM Press, New York (2002)
7. Kung, Y.-S., Shu, G.-S.: Design and implementation of a control IC for vertical articulated robot arm using SOPC technology. In: IEEE International Conference on Mechatronics, pp. 532–536 (2006)
8. Zammattio, S.: SOPC Builder, a Novel Design Methodology for IP Integration. In: Proceedings of International Symposium on System on Chip, p. 37 (2005)

A Study on the Basic Social Network Features of City Sports Population in Henan Province

Mei-ling Duan

Sports Institute Athletics Department, Zhengzhou Childhood education normal school
450000 Zhengzhou, Henan, China
duan-meiling@sohu.com

Abstract. Resorting to literature, questionnaire, consultation and logical analysis, the author of this paper gives a profound research into the scale, density, heterogeneity and convergence of the basic social network features of city sports population in Henan Province. The results show that its features lie in small scale, deep density, high convergence and low heterogeneity. The study aims to explore the strategy and methods of developing city sports population in Henan province so as to speed up the steps of transforming Henan from a big sports province to a strong sports province.

Keywords: city sports population, social network, basic features.

1 Introduction

City Sports refers to the participation in sports activities for the population of the common signs of city social groups composed of individuals, and rooted in the social network of the largest among the special groups. Therefore, as a special social group in a different city, sports classes in the population because of their social network relations will also present the characteristics of the different sectors involved. With the diversity of changes in social strata, which will bring all levels of participation in physical activity needs of the diversity and uniqueness, highlights the status and resources of all different sectors, the population participate in sports activities will also be showing a different social network characteristics. Some of the traditional development strategies for social sports, such as executive orders, and political propaganda will become increasingly difficult to work, and not conducive to the development of sports in our society and the enhancement of the national constitution. Therefore, how to adapt to the hierarchical class structure at this stage of development status and the possibility of future change, explore strategies to rapidly improve sports, development of sports in our society sustainable development strategy has become a serious problem facing. Based on sociological theories and methods of sports population in Henan Province, basic characteristics of social networks, targeted to explore the sports population in Henan Province to develop strategies and methods in Henan Province, to help the competent department to lay down the laws and regulations related to social sports, and policies to guide the sustainable development of social sports reference in practice, to accelerate Henan province into the Sport Pace Province.

L. Qi (Ed.): PDCN 2010, CCIS 137, pp. 85–91, 2011.
© Springer-Verlag Berlin Heidelberg 2011

2 Analysis on Sports Population Size of Social Network in Henan Province

Size of social network characteristics constitute the basic elements of social networks, constituting a social network refers to the number of members, each member often "self" concept to title. Previous studies have shown that the scale is a measure of individual social networks, having an important indicator of social capital. A person in society has a larger social network; he (she) has the more extensive social capital, the more likely to occupy the dominant position of social interaction [1]. This paper analyzes urban sports population in Henan Province is the network size and self in the past six months the total number of sports activities. Projects depend on the American General Social Survey question, using the social network research in the nomination of the widespread use of measurement techniques, following up to 5 nominated members of the international practice of social networks on the Henan Province sports population size of social network analysis.

In some cases, it is the Contact Volume Editor that checks all the pdfs. In such cases, the authors are not involved in the checking phase.

Table 1. The size of social network sports population in Henan Province (N = 723)

Network size (number)	0	1	2	3	4	5
Network size (member)	12	33	98	355	161	64
%	2	4.6	13.6	49.1	22	8.7
Average (member)				3.17		
Standard deviation				1.89		

Note: The standard deviation is the deviation from the mean distance of the average of the data; it reflects the dispersion of a database. A larger standard deviation represents most of the value and the average difference between the larger, and vice versa closer to average. Social network size of sports population in Henan Province was 1.89 standard deviations, which indicates more reliable values.

The data of Table 1 analyzed according to Henan city the size of social network sports population is 3.17 people on average, in the past six months, each member sported with 3.17 member of the network members on average, only 2% of the members did not join with any other members of the sports activities, participating in a social network sports more than the membership rate is 98%. However, in other provinces and cities, because there is no social network sports population scale of the related research, cannot compare the real position of the sports population in Henan Province the size of social networks. But, compared with the size of our network of 314 city residents [2], average of only 0.03 more. Analysis of the fitness from sports and social functions explained the sports population size of social network in Henan Province is relatively small.

3 Analysis on Sports Population Density of Social Network in Henan Province

3.1 Sports in Henan Province Population and the Close Degree of Network Members

Table 2 can be analyzed sports population in Henan Province self social networks closely with network members, the average level was 94.7%, noting the close degree of discussion network very high, From the first network to the fifth member, the closeness is 98.5%, respectively, 95.6%, 94.5%, 85.3% and 81.2%. With the nomination of the delay order, the closeness has a downward trend. However, the percentage of the overall closeness is maintained over ninety percent, saying Henan Province sports population density of social networks more closely, is a high-density groups, with high density. Community participate in sports activities is more than individual alone, and in most cases a majority of people involved, to build some relationships of group activities by physical exercise, and making friends during the exchange of information, gaining friendship from the group. Individual sports groups could get the pleasure of the mind, by body exercise, people wanted to get more friendship and support in the circle of friends, network members knew each circle , the proportion of relatively high density of network members is relatively high.

Table 2. The close degree between sports self population in Henan Province and network members

	The first members of the network	The second members of the network	The third members of the network	The fourth members of the network	The fifth members of the network	Sample totle (%)
Close number	700	648	548	192	52	
Close degree (%)	98.5	95.6	94.5	85.3	81.2	94.7
N	711	678	580	225	64	2258

3.2 The Age Heterogeneity of the Social Network Sports Population in Henan Province

In the sports index analysis of the age heterogeneity of the sports population in Henan Province , based on sociological theory, the index is defined as the age several levels , less than 5 years ,5-10 years (not including 10 years) ,10-15 years (not including 15 years), more than 15 years, to analyze the social network differences between the age heterogeneities.

Table 3. The age heterogeneity of the social network sports population in Henan Province

	%	Average	Standard Deviation	N
Age Heterogeneity				
< 5	46.3	7.67	6.98	678
5—10 (not including 10)	20.1			
10—15 (not including 15)	14.7			
> 15	18.9			

According to Table 3, 46.3% of the age difference between members of the network is less than 5 years, belongs to the same age group, 5-10 years accounted for 20.1%, Accounted for more than 15 years, 18.9%, the average age difference of the network members is 7.67 years, the age heterogeneous of the social networks sports population in Henan Province are less. In sports, members of the network's activities were in the common space, jointly participated in sports activities, freely chose their favorite sports, manner and time, and depended on their own hobbies and interests, Freedom of autonomy, relaxed and happy to engage in physical activity. Network members of different ages together participated in sports as a common interest activity to get the fun from the physical exercise. Age is not the baffle that stopped people to participate in sports activities, people of all ages can go together due to common love of sports.

3.3   The Class Heterogeneity of the Social Network Sports Population in Henan Province

Note: In a hierarchical analysis of the heterogeneity index, according to sociological stratification theory, the segments of the population in Henan Province is divided into professional sports administration class, ordinary white-collar, small employer class and the working class. The same class is "0"; the different class is "1".

According to Table 4, in the social discussion network of the sports population in Henan Province, With 68.9% of the class status of network members was the same, Only 14.8% of the members of the network was completely different class status, the network class heterogeneity average was 0.34, the standard deviation is 0.39, from the class heterogeneity, we can clearly saw that sports population in Henan Province are inclined to self-class status discuss issues that are important for their own with the same class people, the heterogeneity index level was relatively low. Because of the different class structure, in particular, the choice of sports activities exist very big difference among the various sectors. Only on the economic base could a certain number of sports participate, such as golf, tennis and other projects, requiring certain equipment and sites [4]. People to participate in various sports activities seemed to be a symbol of their identities and social status symbols, most of the members with training and self-class members were the same or similar income.

Table 4. The class heterogeneity of the social network sports population in Henan Province

	%	Average	Standard Deviation (S.D.)	N
Class heterogeneity				
0	68.9			
0.01—0.99	16.3	0.34	0.39	678
1	14.8			

4   Sports Population in Henan Province Convergence of Social Networks

Convergence of social networks in this paper refers specifically to the similarities between selves and members of other social network in certain social characteristics.

Most people tend to contact with persons of similar background [5], or of similar level of education, age. So the more similar, people are more likely to communicate. Network heterogeneity and network convergence, the two interrelated indicators for measurement of social network characteristics and differences, but they are from different areas to reflect the structure of social networks. This paper analyzes the social network indicators that reflect the heterogeneity of the social network between members, not including the self, as well as the degree of similarities and differences on some indicators in the social network. The heterogeneity of indicators measures the difference between social network members. The convergence of social network index is a comparison between network members and selves in terms of social characteristics and differences in degrees. The indicators of convergence in this paper analyzed ruled out the cases of network size 0.

4.1 Convergence on Gender for the Social Network Sports Population in Henan Province

In this study, it takes the percentage of members with the same gender in the total network as the index to study gender convergence. Completely different gender is set as 0, completely same gender is 100, divided into more than a few indicators.

Sports population in Henan Province gender convergence of social networks can be seen from the table, the percentage of the gender convergence between the selves and members of the network in our analysis accounted for 67.5% of all the samples, the percentage can reach 36.4% between selves and all members involved in the discussion, only 9.1% completely different in gender, indicating that in sports activities, sports population in Henan Province and numbers of the member of the same gender in the participation of sports are high. The people like to participate in the sports with the persons sharing the same gender. So it can be known that the network discussed at present is one with the higher convergence of gender.

Table 5. Sports population in Henan Province convergence of social networks

Variable	%	Average	Standard Deviation (S.D.)	N
convergence on gender				
0	9.1			
1—99	54.5	67.5	32.1	711
100	36.4			

4.2 Convergence on Age for Social Network Sports Population in Henan Province

In the analysis of sports population of Henan Province convergence of social network we set the percentage of the members five years older or younger than the investigated in the total number as the indicator of the study.

Table 6. Convergence on age for Social Network sports population in Henan Province

	%	Standard Deviation (S.D.)	N
Convergence on age	60.5		
Five years younger than the self	18.4	32.6	711
Five years older than the self	21.1		

Data in the table 6 shows that age of convergence for the sports population in cites of Henan province social network is relatively high, with 60.5% of the network members in this range of age, the members five years younger than the self in the network accounted for 18.4%, and 5 years older than the self accounted for 21.1%, indicating that convergence on age In the study is high. It show that members sharing similar ages hope to participate in the similar sports as their hobbies.

4.3. Convergence on Class for Social Network Sports Population in Henan Province

According to research needs and Professor Zhang Wenhong's class classification methods; this paper divides the class into the following categories in rank, that is, the level of professional executive management, small employer class, ordinary white-collar and working class.

Table 7. Convergence on class for Social Network sports population in Henan Province

	%	Standard Deviation (S.D.)	N
convergence on class	57.9		
With higher class	25.2	39.7	711
With lower class	16.9		

The table 7 shows that the percentage of convergence on class for Social Network sports population in Henan Province is 57.9%, the members with higher status than the self accounted for 25.2%, with lower status than the self accounted for 16.9%. it shows that the people in this province have a strong class tendency when they choose the members in the participation of sports. Therefore, after the analysis of these indicators, it shows that the convergence on age, gender and class is very high. It indicates the constitution of the social network on the sport population in Henan Province has clear group boundaries. There is a strong tendency to self-selection, with characteristics of high convergence.

According to the model of opportunities and constraints of social interaction theory, people generally tend to develop close relationships with the people showing similar social characteristics as themselves, attitudes, status, behavior and beliefs promote people with similar social status to form a close relationship. The individuals with different attitude, status, behavior and beliefs are not likely to the form the close relationship in the later contact [6]. In sports activities, activities for the professional administrative class and white-collar class are not only for their own exercise, but for the pursuit of the enjoyment of life, and the personalized service, highlighting the identity and status. They are mostly involved in the sports in the form of individuals or small groups, such as tennis, badminton, golf, yoga, swimming, etc., but for large groups and the fiercely competitive activities, that are reluctant to participate. With a good economic condition and more rest time, so they prefer to participate in the sport with high consumption. The members in the network share the similar economic condition and interests, so they have more exercise time together. And the social network convergence is high [7]. For the working class, due to pressure from family and work, so they tend to choose some sports with short time and less money, selecting sports more affordable and the main purpose is to exercise the body, enhance physical fitness. Entertainment requirements are reduced, and the exchange with the members in upper classes is few. With the similar interest in the popular recreational sport, the people like to participate in physical exercise with similar status and background, which is the main reason for the high convergence in social network.

5   Conclusion

Social network of the sports population in Henan Province is relatively small, which did not reflect the sport's functions of social communication and fitness. Social network of the sports population in Henan Province has the characteristics of high density, mainly in the high frequency of interaction and the long duration of the relationship. Social network of the sports population in Henan Province has characteristics of low heterogeneity, mainly in the heterogeneity of gender, class and the age. Social network of the sports population in Henan Province has the characteristics of high convergence, mainly in high convergence of gender, class and the age.

Acknowledgments. Fund Program: Philosophy and Social Sciences in 2008 Planning Project in Henan Province, "City Sports in Henan Province Population characteristics and composition of the social network model of" (2008CTY004).

References

1. Lin, N.: Social Capital: A Theory of Social Structure and Action. Cambridge University Press, Cambridge (2001)
2. Chang, W.-H.: China City Ierarchical Structures and Social Network, pp. 77–79. Shanghai People's Publishing House (2006)
3. Granovetter, M.: The Strength of Weak Ties. American Journal of Sociology (8), 1360–1380 (1973)
4. Zhu, R., Wang, W.-L.: Ganzhou City Urban Sports Population Structure Layered Development Countermeasures. Chifeng University Journal (Natural Science Edition) 25(11), 94–95
5. Blau: Inequality and Heterogeneity. The Free Press, New York (1977)
6. Chang, W.-H., Li, P.-L., Ruan, D.-Q.: City Residents of Social Network Class Composition. Sociology Research 6, 1–10 (2004)
7. Tang, G.-J.: Research on the Perspective under Social Stratification of Urban Sports Population Structure and Activity Characteristics. Beijing Sport University Journals 31(9), 1185–1187 (2008)

The Brief Explanation of Physical Violence in Sociology

Jinliang Chen

Faculty of Physical Education of Henan Business College, Zhengzhou,
Henan province, China
7717731@qq.com

Abstract. With the development of our society, great changes have taken place in the way of people's work and life, sports are becoming more and more important. The sport as a part of culture and education, it's value can not be ignored. It can enrich people's life, improve the quality of life, additionally, their have great values in education, fitness and entertainment. Stadium Sports violence is a very troublesome social problem in the current world, to the pursuit of the harmonious development of human society, casting a shadow over the sports. This article will analyze the causes of violence from the sociological point, to provide a theoretical basis to the solution to the problem of violence.

Keywords: sociology, physical violence, theoretical basis.

1 Introduction

As our country in social transition, sports management system needs to be improved, to some extent, it is contributed to the spread of violence in sports stadium. Social psychologists define it in different ways, it is reflected mainly in the intent rather than results. From a sociological analysis, the physical violence is a concrete manifestation of different forms of conflict, not only a cultural phenomenon, but also a complex social phenomenon, having deep social roots, so their analysis from a sociological point is necessary.

2 Stadium Sports Violence and Classification

2.1 The Concept of Violence in Sports Stadium

Social psychologists define violence in different ways. One is that violence is any action or behavior to hurt the others. Under this definition, the results of actions are important. Another view is that violence is mainly reflected in the intentions of actions rather than the results [3]. Strictly speaking, violence is the intentional actions or behavior to injury any others. Performances of sports stadium violence happen between the competitors, the audiences, the players and referees, spectators and referees and sports officials and some other violent incidents in or outside the arenas. A western football stadium has more than one record that more than a hundred audiences' deaths caused by violence, besides athletes are shot dead and injury rivals.

L. Qi (Ed.): PDCN 2010, CCIS 137, pp. 92–96, 2011.

2.2 Physical Violence Is a Manifestation to Different forms of Conflicts, Violence Can Be Divided into Constructive and Destructive Violence

Constructive violence is the inherent properties of sports, is a special form of conflict, is a ritual war, is a safety valve for social conflicts, is regarded as the outbreak of aggression and aggressive behavior and reduce some other systems of society conflicts, not only meet the needs of the social system, but also avoid a large-scale war, conducive violence is good to social development, it appears as the emergence of sports, it's the inherent nature of sport interior.

Destructive violence is "alienation" to competitive, has the feature of modern sport of violence, it can be divided into sports violence, violence in the stands and mixed s violence.

There are both links and differences between them. Both they are behaviors and phenomena caused by sports and the results will bring varying degrees of pain and injury, resulting in varying degrees of conflict or even be in conflict. They often happen at the same time, destructive violent sports can be seen as the results of further development of the constructive [4].

3 The Reality Reflects of Violence in Sports Stadium

3.1 Physical Violence Court Forms

Aggressive behavior in movements can occur between athletes, appear in the athletes and coaches, referees, or between coaches and coaches, between coaches and referees, but also in the audience and the audience, viewers and athletes, the audience or the audience and judges. For example, in the sports arena often occur some major fans riot. Football is very popular in our country. Because the characteristics of the project itself (direct contact with the body, the opponents), leading to aggressive behavior in some football matches often, and caused some serious adverse effects.

3.2 The Attack Strength of Different Sports Is Different (as Table 1)

As we all known: the attack strength of contact sport is stronger than non-contact sport; Both are contact sports but different in projects, such as boxing is more offensive than football, football is more aggressive than basketball.

Table 1. Different levels of aggressive sports classification

level	Direct against	Limited attack	Indirect attack	For objects of attacks	Attack rarely
For example	boxing	football	tennis	golf	Figure skating
For example	rugby	basketball	volleyball	track and field	athletics gymnastics

4   Causes of Stadium Sports Violence

4.1   Physical Violence Courts Have a Definite Link of the Dominant Values of the Entire Community

Modern society, the pursuit of success is the dream of community members, as long as success, one can do at all costs and by all means. Sports as an integral part of society will be inevitably caused by the impact of these values. The professional, commercial of competitive sport is exacerbated by the pursuit of money and interest. Talking about sports, people pay more attention to sports results and sports stars who shine, and many sports stars are especially pursued by young people, even regarded as a hero. Winner takes all, and the arena likes to be a battlefield. Take the football World Cup for example, dozens of teams like dozens of Armies, winners like to be a hero and the fans cheer like thunder drums which can be sound everywhere and surrounded by flowers; but losers are desolately different. Community also give special love to heroes, once get a champion, fame and fortune will come one after another, and even can became a film star, business giant quickly. In this social environment, sports have become a successful dream stage, the instrumental value of sports is above the entertainment value, more and more away from its origin. Utilitarian is dominant in the current society, the spiritual value of sports is ignored, doctrine championship become the dominant, athletes pursue to success at all means. Therefore, sports stadium violence appear between the athletes, athletes and coaches, referees, or between coaches and coaches, between coaches and referees, but also in the audience and the audience, and viewers and athletes, spectators with the coach or between the audience and judges.

4.2   China Is in the Social Transition, the Sports Management Systems Are to Be Improved

At present, we are in the transition period, there are some abnormal phenomena in sports management, sports industry, operational, and cultural publicity, resulting in sports team do secret operations of the game, gambling, match-fixing in pursuit of the greatest professional economic interests, the conflicts are intensified between the team, the fans and the referees, which have become the incentive causes for violent sports stadium. The media expand the economic benefits of the expansion of sports ,at the same time, they also contribute to the spread of violence in sports stadium, especially the young people growing up in this environment, which has become commonplace and no longer harbor disgust, they watch the violence not only for the fun , while in stimulating atmosphere of the stadium, if the performance of athletes and the results cause their dissatisfaction, they often do aggressive behavior, personally contribute to and participate in violence. Of course, these are problems in the development, with the gradual improvement of our society, these problems will be effectively addressed.

4.3   To Establish Good Social Values

In the Contemporary Athletics development process, professional and commercialization to sports bring vitality and vigor, athletes are also faced with the stark effect of interest and money, the inner world is difficult to balance, so in sports training players must be starting from themselves and strict on themselves in order to improve small environment to optimize the social environment, to deal with several complex problems in the real-life. While competitive social value lies in the individual, collective and State interests linked to the athletic activities, so that the player is in a kind of social tensions. Sports competition is the epitome of social competition and sports, through sports training and competition to motivate their hardworking, cultivating good psychological, moraquality and spirit of cooperation, such as compliance with the rules can develop their law behavior norms.

4.4 To Establish a Good Relationship between the Individual and Group

In the Competitive sports, coaches, athletes, referees, sports officials and spectators all play different roles, they have own values with competitive, therefore in competitive, individual and group for values and behaviour of different produce conflict of roles, how to solve a variety of social conflicts subsided, various social groups of discontent, avoid contradictions of repression and concentrated, is also a problem faced by the athletes. Athletes are special groups of, is the important social role, they are the subject role of competitive sports, is the creator of sports culture, but also the human fundamental values of the load. So for athletic groups you want to learn the sport do appropriate social roles that individual in sports or exercise compatible with groups, are met, the coordination of various relationships. This relationship can coordinate the role of mutual support and mutual trust, promote the healthy development of the athlete's personality, improve players ' pride and consciousness. If an athlete can well handled relationships with leader, coach, teammates, opponents, magistrate audience, and have well habits with sincere cooperation and fair competition, with good interpersonal applied forces reduce and prevent the occurrence of violent behavior.

4.5 To Strengthen the Education of Ideological and Discipline

Atheltes' training, in order to get good grades, is almost closed, but this is adversary for them psychologically. The Athlete adminstraters should encourage athletes to participate in social activities in order to integrat into society and achieve social changes. Since sports have been market-oriented, athletes can not be required being completely secluded. When athletes have some problems, it is primarily to utilize criticized education, taking advantage of our traditional ideological and political work, making more communications, and adopting more flexible approach instead of tauting and castigation. Only throught making a rational tolerance and laying empathy can solve the athletes' real problems.

4.6 Improve the Level of Athletes' Quality

Enhancing the cultural quality of athletes can not only improving their intellectual level but also help them make a higher vision, a broader mind and maintain a better state when participate in momentous game. The impact of scientific and cultural knowledge can be deep into the athlete's values and enable athletes being diligent in thinking, being of good sentiment, which can promote their values changing and thus change the behavior of athletes and their life.

4.7 Being Actively Adapt to the Mass Media and Public Opinion

Mass media and public opinion are with the timeliness and sensitivity, can provide athletes with information and knowledge and attract social attention, influence attitudes and behavior of athletes, impact the psychological state before and after the game. But when the media and public opinion more than a certain limit, it will make athletes over-excited or extremely depressed. If improperly handled this may lead to serious consequences. How to correctly judge and make the athletes adapted to the media and public opinion, reduce stress and prevent violence remain a major problem in sports.

References

[1] Lu, Y.: Chinese sports sociology. Beijing sport university press, Beijing (2000)
[2] Wang, R.: Athletes of offensive behavior. In: Zhang, W., Ren, W. (eds.) Advances in Sport Psychology. Higher education press, Beijing (November 2000)
[3] Zhu, B. (ed.): Principles and applications of Sport Psychology. East China institute of chemical press, Shaihai (1992)
[4] Shi, Y.: China football spectator violence situation and issues. Beijing Sport University Journals 27(8), 1013–1015 (2004)

On the Disciplinary Attributes, Characteristics and Scope of Sports Economics

Wu Xudong

Department of Physical Education,
Zhengzhou University,
450001 Zhengzhou, Henan
its4ad@gmail.com

Abstract. Sports economics is a new discipline. It has developed in our country for only over a decade. The discussion about its basic concept has never been stopped. Its primary task is to get to understand the disciplinary attributes, characteristics and scope of this discipline. This paper tries to clarify its disciplinary attributes, highlights its disciplinary characteristics and defines its research scope, combined with the research results of relevant scholars and related disciplines.

Keywords: Discipline, Disciplinary attributes, Interdisciplinary subjects, Sports Economics.

1 Introduction

"Subject" is an English word "discipline" which, on the one hand, refers to the classification of knowledge and the subject of study, on the other hand, means the cultivation of people. When "discipline" is translated into "subject", its meanings of other aspects are neglected.

From the angle of transferring knowledge and education teaching, discipline means "teaching subject" which is the subject of teaching and the one of learning; from the angle of knowledge of production and research of learning, it indicates the branch of learning which is a branch of science and the classification of knowledge; from the angle of college teaching and research organization, it is an academic organization which is engaged in teaching and research.

Angles once had a brilliant exposition about the disciplinary attribute," Every discipline is to analyses some specific athletic forms, or a series of interrelated and interchangeable athletic forms, so its classification is the one based on inherent orders."

Every disciple experiences a development process, which is from birth to growth to maturity, and then to becoming a new branch after mixing with other branches of discipline or based on the original discipline. Sports economics, as a new inter-disciplinary subject, appeared in the early 1990s and its discipline system has gradually been established and perfected until now. The establishment of discipline system of sports economics will greatly enhance the discipline in turn. The development goal becomes clear and definite. The research of economics experts and sports science

L. Qi (Ed.): PDCN 2010, CCIS 137, pp. 97–103, 2011.

experts will focus on the discipline. The crossing research activities will play an active role in promoting the development of the discipline system.

2 Birth of Sports Economics

After the Second World War, the international situations are easing; science and technology is rapid progressing; the productivity levels of developed countries are rapidly improved; the national economy continues to grow, which all stimulate the vigorous development of the sports and thus promote the birth and development of sports economics.

2.1 File Social and Economic Development Caused the Birth of Sports Economics

As society and economy developing, the improvement of living standards of people, the increase of leisure time and changes of lifestyle cause the significant changes of people's social demand structure. Sports population is increasing. People's attention to sports becomes higher and higher. The economic problems in the sports fields are becoming increasingly serious, which attract the attention of people.

2.2 Commercialization of Athletic Sports Promotes the Development of Sports Economics

There is a close connection between the birth and development of problems in sports economics and commercialization of athletic sports. Olympic professionalism and the penetration of commercial factors have raised professional sports to a high position. The position of sports as an industry also gets laid.

2.3 Sports Consumption Demands Are Being Increased, Which Propel the Development of Sports Economics

With the enhancement of sports consciousness of people, the increase of sports population, sports consumption demand of people becomes rapidly increased, esp. demand of sports service that is beneficial to the development of sports industry. That the sports industry plays an more important role in the national economy and gets economic benefits attracts people's attention, which propel the development of sports economics.

3 Disciplinary Attribute Discrimination of Sports Economics

Sports economics faces an important question since its birth, which is its disciplinary attribute discrimination. It restricts the development direction of sports economical discipline. If the contents of sports economics are too many, too miscellaneous, it is easy to lead to generalization of its academic research that makes it lose its attribute; conversely, it also was disadvantageous to its prosperity and development. So, how to define the disciplinary attribute of sports economics becomes a big question. Only establishing its scientific and reasonable academic attribute, its research direction and research content will have adequate theoretical basis.

3.1 Three Opinions of Disciplinary Attribute of Sports Economics

Economic subject attribute. Economics includes a lot of subjects, which generally can be divided into two levels: theoretical economics and applied economics. Theoretical economics talks about its basic concept, theories and general rule of movement and development of economy that provide basic theories to every economics branch. Applied economics is mainly to apply its relevant basic theories to making a study on economic activities in every unit of national economy and every professional field, or to analyzing the economic and social effectiveness in non-economic fields. It includes every economics discipline which has sector economics such as industrial economics, educational economics, and agricultural economics, and has professional economics, such as, population economics, labor economics, ecological economics, which all are based on the theoretical economics and are branches in the economics system.

Sports economics is a branch of economics. People in support of this think it is a sector economics like educational economics and agricultural economics whose economics attribute will become obvious with the development of discipline of sports economics.

Sport subject attribute. In 1992, classification and code of disciplines in the People's Republic of China national standards regards sports as a first-level discipline and add it to humanities and social science, and economics sports as one of its 12 second-level disciplines and adds it to sport humanistic sociology. In the teaching practices, people always add sports economics to the category of sports science. It was because it first appeared in sports field. The first scholar who studied sports economics was born in sports field. The groups of scholars form the academic communities among sports colleges and relevant sports scientific research personnel, and organize the industry societies. So, it is generally believed that it has sport subject attribute.

Interdisciplinary attributes. People who hold this opinion think that sports economics is a comprehensive product of sports science and economics disciplines. It is an interdisciplinary subject. It proposes not to be eager to put it to a particular subject at the present, which is good to absorb research results of other subjects. Making a multi-sided study on sports economics is beneficial to its growing at the early stage.

3.2 Disciplinary Attributes of Sports Economics

Then, what is the disciplinary attribute of sports economics? The author thinks that, to answer this question, first must know what standards to classify disciplines and what relations among every classification. There are many standards to classify the nature of disciplines. But there are two main: one classification is according to the scientific research objects; the other is according to the scientific research methods. According to what standards is the disciplinary attribute of sports economics as a new subject classified? Obviously, it is scientific to use research objects as a standard to talk about the disciplinary attribute of sports economics, because it is based on the categories and levels of objective things that is good to clear the position and level of sports economics in the disciplinary system.

Question one about the attributes of sports economics. Whether sports economics is regarded as a branch of sports science or a branch of economic science is vague, both of which can not reveal the disciplinary attribute of sports economics. It is necessary to deeply explore its disciplinary attribute according to the development of the discipline and its internal characteristics.

Question two about the attributes of sports economics. Sports economics is an interdisciplinary subject. It can be understood from two aspects: (1) sports economics is on sports economy form the angle of economics. So, to know its nature, we must study and grasp the related knowledge of sports science, such as, sports club, athletic training, sports products; at the same time, to introduce its concept, category and to avoid turning sports economics research into abstract concepts, we must explain it by using materials provided by sports science to make a organic combination between theories and practices, and between history and logic. So sports economics not only includes the content of sports science, but also the one of economics science. (2) Many scientific researches on sports economics are purely difficult to resolve such questions as the supply and demand of sports market and sports consumption behaviour which need many subjects together. But the key question is whether disciplinary subject becomes the main and only classification of sports economics? I don't think so. First, the disciplinary subject is only one research method in many situations. Inter by itself is not the purpose. But our goal is to resolve the question, e.g. mathematical economics which uses mathematics method to describe economics theory. So, we can not go to extremes in thinking about this. Second, various disciplines of interdisciplinary science have the same important.

Position in many situations. One side is the main, but the others are secondary. Third, the interdisciplinary subject is not putting two subjects together mechanically, but extrapolating them and understanding them from the angle of multiple disciplines. So, about disciplinary attribute of sports economics, we should think of it as interdisciplinary subject, but should not be content with it.

Conclusion of the attributes of sports economics. Although sports economics is an interdisciplinary subject, it is mainly an economics science and a branch of economics. Because, first, the position of every aspect that crosses with others inside the sports economics is unbalanced, and the economic problems in sports fields are its main research objects. Second, the research objects and methods of sports economics are almost same with general economics. Third, establishing sports economics as a branch of economics is fit in with development needs of sports economics.

The important significance to establish the attributes of sports economics
Establishing the attribute of sports economics has the important significance. First, it is good to determine the main task of sports economics which is the study of movement essence of sports economics and its development rule. Second, it is good to select its main logic research method. Third, it is good to establish discipline system of sports economics.

4   The Basic Characteristics of Sports Economics

Sports economics is a new discipline. Its main characteristics are three following:

4.1   The Sports Characteristic

Compared with other economics science, sports economics mainly discusses about the relationship between sports and economics, and about how limited sports resources is effectively allocated. Sports this special cultural phenomenon has the inseparable connection with social and economic phenomenon. Economy is the foundation of sports emergence and development, whose development restricts sports development. At the same time, the scale and development level of sports can reflect the status and level of economic development.

Sports economics is an art which discusses about how limited sports resources is effectively allocated and also about dealing with the problems in sports field by using the knowledge of economics, which fully shows the sports characteristic, that is, we cannot mechanically apply the term and regularity in the economic field to the sports field. We should discern economic law and economic concepts to clarify its economic phenomenon according to the characteristics of the sports fields and combining with practices.

4.2   The Theoretical Characteristic

Although sports economics is different form general economics, they have the same characteristics. They are theoretical sciences. So, sports economics are a series of concepts, categories and laws in forms. It can explain and predict sports economic phenomenon in contents. If sports economics has no theoretical characteristic, it is difficult to understand the essence of sports economy movement, which is determined by its research content and task.

It is alleged that the most important of sports economics is to strengthen practical problems, because theoretical research examines nonsense. This point is one-sided. Research on practical problems is really important, but it cannot replace the theoretical research which can provide analysis tools and theoretical bases for practical problems.

4.3   The Empirical Characteristic

Sports economics stresses objectivity and empirical characteristic. It deals with such problems as, what characteristics objective things have, what are their operation mechanism and why they operate like this. It should not discuss how to do it only from the angle of some standard.

5   Research Scope of Sports Economics

Sports economics should answer three questions: why sports have economic value? How to effectively allocate the sports resources? How to effectively operate sports organizations? We talk about research scope of sports economics around these three questions.

5.1 Why Sports Have Economic Value?

To answer this question, we will start from the relation between sports and economics, dealing with sports products and intangible assets and with how sports raise the consumption level of people.

Sports have the irreplaceable value in two aspects that are to enhance human capital and to improve consumption level and skills. "Sports forms human capital" and "sports improve consumption level and skills" are double-point links where sports have the relation to social and economic questions. These two themes are the basic premises, on which other questions arise.

5.2 How to Effectively Allocate the Sports Resources?

Talking about resources, we should think of the optimal market allocation problem. Sports products not only have the non-competitive, non-exclusive characteristics of public products, also have the competitive and exclusive characteristics of private products. Sports are a converged product that converges the factors of public products and the ones of private products.

The question of sports economics starts from the contradiction between the ultimate purpose of sports and its living conditions. This living condition refers to the resource condition that can realize economic value and ultimate purpose. Whether individuals make sports activities, or society or government develop sports career and sports industry, they will consider cost problem which is something that people will quit and invest in order to wake up sports activities and society and to develop sports industry and sports career.

That is to say, sports needs cost, which is the basic premise of how to provide adequate resources for sports.

5.3 How to Effectively Operate Sports Organizations?

Sports organizations are of the government or folk. The movement process of sports organizations has deeper characteristics of economics. The management behaviour closely related to market begins to appear in many links of the operation and management of sports organizations. The management of sports organizations becomes an effective method to realize economic value and goals.

6 Conclusion

As sports economics is a new discipline, there are many different opinions about its disciplinary attribute and research scope. It has not yet formed a complete theoretical system. So, its reflection and discussion may promote its theoretical research and applied research in our country.

References

1. Marx, K., Engles, F.: Marx Engels complete works, p. 593. People's Publishing House, Beijing (1971)
2. Zhong, T.: Introduction to sports economics. Fudan University Press, Shanghai (2007)
3. Cong, H.: Sports economics. Higher Education Press, Beijing (2004)
4. Kong, H.: Reasons of the reconstruction of college academic structure
5. Hu, J.: Innovation of discipline organizations, pp. 243–244. Zhejiang University Press, Hangzhou (2001)

Formulation and Application of Evaluation Questionnaire on Teaching Quality of Sports Colleges Track and Field Course

Shuyu Xia

Sports Institute Athletics Department, Physical Education College of Zhengzhou University
Zhengzhou, Henan, China
xs19750207@yahoo.com.cn

Abstract. Higher requests have been put forwagd to teacher's quality and sports teaching quality in order to adapt to cultivating the 21st century sports talents needs, and to cultivate high-quality teachers for primary and secondary schools. To establish a complete system of sports colleges track and field course, fifteen variables and seven factors are selected by means of mathematical statistics and analytical hierarchy process etc. and an evaluation questionnaire on sports colleges track and field course is worked out.

Keywords: Evaluation questionnaire, sports colleges track and field course, teaching quality.

1 Introduction

Sports colleges' track and field course is an important constituent of sports education in our country. It is the main target and primary task of P.E. to cultivate talents adapting to the 21st century. Along with the deepening of teaching reformation, primary secondary schools are comprehensively implement the *Physical Education (and Health) Curriculum Standard* which puts forward higher request to the teachers' quality and school's teaching management level in many aspects, such as basic idea and design idea of course, choice of content of teaching target and course, teaching advice, teaching evaluation, and utilization and development of curriculum resource. It is a current problem to be solved for us how to improve the teaching quality of track and field course, to build a scientific evaluation system.

2 Research Objects and Methods

Interviews with Experts. Consult and communicate with experts by means of Face-to-face interviews, telephone interviews and network video etc. Among professor: 47%; Associate professor: 53%.

L. Qi (Ed.): PDCN 2010, CCIS 137, pp. 104–109, 2011.

Questionnaire
Consult massively the relevant materials and monographs, and to some experts, then a questionnaire was worked out and some tests was done to make sure of its effectiveness and reliability, they were found to accord with the requirements. 100 copies of investigating questionnaires were issued to the experts and scholars in athletics teaching (given in the Appendix), and recycled 92 copies of that, the recovery is 92%. Among which 12 copies were eliminated because of invalidity. 80 copies are valid, and the valid recovery is 96.74%. All of these comply with the requirement of scientific research, and can reflect the evaluation identity of experts and scholars about athletics teaching nowadays.

Mathematic Statistics. After the questionnaires were recycled, some processing work on them was done, and the data was calculated statistically and analyzed mathematically with SPSS software.

3 Results and Analysis

3.1 Selection of the Index Influencing the Athletics Teaching Quality

First, according to the basic laws of athletic teaching, consult the relevant materials about the theories of teaching on class, track and field course, sports curriculum design and the structure of track and field course, select the index that may influence teaching quality and reflect the status of bilateral activity of teaching and learning, classify them into five degrees, they are "very important, fundamental important, important, unimportant, very unimportant". The value of them are 5, 4, 3, 2, 1 relatively. Finish the questionnaires statistically and select the indexes that larger than 4.

Relatively they are X1--teacher's lesson plans, X2--preparation of field and sports facilities, X3--teacher's apperance, X4—exercise, X5—teacher's language arrangement, X6—arrangement and allocate of class time, X7—practice density for students, X8—sports intensity for students, X9—teaching methods, X10—teacher's demonstration skills, X11—arrangement of class, X12—teacher-student interaction, X13—lesson content, X14—the mastering on class for students, X15—realization of teaching goals.

3.2 Analyze the Index of the Factors, Extract the Structures and Name Them

Total Variance Explained

The results of the Factor Extraction are given in Table 1, where C is the Cumulative (%), Com is the Component.

With the Extraction Method: Principal Component Analysis, from Table 1 it is known that seven factors were extracted by means of analysis of the fifteen effective factors, and the contribution rate of the extracted factors reached to 84.22%.

Table 1. Results of the Factor Extraction

Com	Initial Eigen values			Extraction Sums of Squared Loadings			Rotation Sums of Squared Loadings		
	Total	% of Variance	C	Total	% of Variance	C	Total	% of Variance	C
1	3.107	20.715	20.715	3.107	20.715	20.715	2.098	13.987	13.987
2	2.421	16.14	36.855	2.421	16.14	36.855	1.997	13.315	27.302
3	2.022	13.481	50.336	2.022	13.481	50.336	1.915	12.77	40.072
4	1.586	10.573	60.909	1.586	10.573	60.909	1.824	12.157	52.229
5	1.396	9.308	70.217	1.396	9.308	70.217	1.7	11.331	63.56
6	1.187	7.915	78.132	1.187	7.915	78.132	1.632	10.877	74.437
7	0.913	6.09	84.222	0.913	6.09	84.222	1.468	9.785	84.222
8	0.779	5.197	89.418						
9	0.446	2.975	92.394						
10	0.436	2.91	95.303						
11	0.309	2.057	97.36						
12	0.151	1.008	98.368						
13	0.134	0.893	99.26						
14	6.68E-02	0.446	99.706						
15	4.41E-02	0.294	100						

Component Score Coefficient Matrix

Table 2. Loading Matrix of Factors (Orthogonal Great Rotation)

	Component						
	1	2	3	4	5	6	7
X1	0.137	0.09	-0.01	0.026	-0.025	0.067	-0.608
X2	-0.048	0.097	-0.034	0.529	-0.01	-0.218	-0.066
X3	0.108	0.051	-0.139	-0.178	0.304	-0.152	0.009
X4	0.06	0.172	-0.06	-0.064	0.077	0.02	0.503
X5	0.174	-0.348	0.115	-0.036	0.006	-0.161	0.124
X6	0.213	0.222	-0.102	0.399	-0.154	0.231	-0.106
X7	-0.114	-0.159	0.034	0.319	0.076	0.113	0.046
X8	-0.558	0.04	0.159	0.099	0.23	0.064	0.126
X9	-0.099	-0.085	-0.073	-0.08	0.018	0.584	-0.059
X10	-0.199	-0.002	0.118	0.027	0.649	0.126	0.055
X11	-0.013	0.056	-0.416	0.101	0.075	0.013	-0.083
X12	0.023	0.477	0.198	0.137	0.071	-0.1	0.137
X13	-0.082	0.165	0.526	0.044	0.193	-0.051	-0.152
X14	0.164	0.184	0.124	0.016	0.124	0.29	0.103
X15	0.228	-0.16	0.127	0.017	0.252	-0.187	0.039

Extraction Method: Principal Component Analysis.
Rotation Method: Varimax with Kaiser Normalization.
Component Scores.
Table 2 shows that seven factors constituting one-class index and contained variable factors can be achieved and named. (See Table 3).

Table 3. Names and Contents of the Factors

Seriel Number	Names of Factors	The contained Variable
Factor 1	Class arrangement	X1,X4
Factor 2	Lesson content	X9
Factor 3	Teacher's appearance	X3,X10
Factor 4	Sports load	X2,X6,X7
Factor 5	Teaching methods	X11,X13
Factor 6	Teaching goals	X5,X12
Factor 7	Preparation before class	X8,X14,X15

3.3 Determination of the Index Weight

The weight means the importance of some index in the evaluation system, that is, under the condition of other factors invariable, the change of the factors influences the evaluation result. The weight of each factor was worked out by means of analytical hierarchy process. (See Table 4).

Table 4. Analysis Table for the Weight of Various Factors

	Factor							
	1	2	3	4	5	6	7	weights
Class arrangement	1.00	2.00	0.17	0.33	3	2	0	0.089
Lesson content	0.50	1.00	0.20	0.5	1	2	0.25	0.066
Teacher's appearance	6.00	5.00	1.00	3	4	5	0.5	0.281
Sports load	3.00	2.00	0.33	1	2	3	0.33	0.130
Teaching methods	0.33	1.00	0.25	0.5	1	1	0.25	0.059
Teaching goals	0.50	0.50	0.20	0.33	1	1	0.25	0.051
Preparation before class	6.00	4.00	2.00	3	4	4	1	0.324

4 Conclusion

The factors influencing the evaluation system of teaching quality of sports colleges track and field course, by experts analysis and questionnaire screening, can be classified into 15 items. The factors by means of factor analysis, were classified into 7 items. Independent and interactive, they promote mutually.

The value of the one-class index influencing the teaching quality of athletics selection specially courses are 7 factors. The order is class arrangement, lesson content, teacher's appearance, sports load, the means of teaching, teaching purpose, and preparation before class etc. Calculate their weights and formulate an evaluation scale for sports collages athletics courses.

References

1. Zhang, Y.: Constructing Efficient Steering Mechanism and Promoting P.E. Teaching Quality, 133 (August 2010)
2. Wu, Y., et al.: New Ideas of College Athletics Teaching Reformation. Journal of Sports Science Research, 88–91 (December 2006)
3. Chen, J., et al.: Physical Statistics, March 17, pp. 213–222. People's Sports Press, Beijing (2002)
4. Education Department. Outline of College Sports Education Athletics Teaching 2002 (2002)
5. Zou, K., et al.: New Ideas of College Athletics Teaching Reformation. Wuhan Sports College Journal, 78–81 (September 2008)
6. Du, J.: Analysis of Characteristics and System Structure of Athletics Teaching Content of Ordinary University. Jilin Sports College Journal, 105–106 (February 2007)

Appendix: Formulation of Evaluation Scale for Sport Colleges' Track and Field Course

Teacher's Name: _____   Title: _____   Unit(School): _____

Class: _____   Number of Students Should Attend:_____

Number of Students Really Attend _____   Date: _____

Evaluation Scale Table for Sports Colleges' Track and field course

Evaluation Index (Weight)	Second-class Index (Weight)	Content of Observation	Scores of Second-class Index	Scores of One-class Index	Note
Preparation before Class (0.324)	Teacher's Lesson Plans (0.48)	The structure of lesson plans complies with the requirements; substantial in content; reasonable assignment			
	Field and Sports Facilities (0.33)	Field and sports facilities; no safe hidden trouble; reasonable assignment			
	Teacher's appearance (0.19)	Teacher' dress meets the requirement and with generous deportment			
Lesson content (0.066)	Lesson content (1)	Familiar to the lesson content, clearly and systemically, and stress the emphasis and difficult points			
Teacher's appearance (0.281)	Language expression (0.43)	Clear explenation.accurate expression; Strict-organized language and standard *Putonghua*			
	Demonstration skills (0.57)	Suitable position,and up to standard; when demonstrating; with various demonstration ways			
Class arrangement (0.089)	Class management (0.46)	Fast and reasonable mobilization of the team,and with safety			
	Arrangement and allotation of class time (0.54)	Compactly-arranged class, Reasonable allotated lesson content, Start and close class timely			
Teaching methods (0.059)	Means of teaching (0.65)	Various and proper teaching methods			
	Teacger-students interaction (0.35)	Be able to arouse students'enthusiasm, and promote each other Harmonious relationship between teacher and students			
Sports load (0.13)	Practice density for students (0.41)	Exercise on class meets to the requirements; Reasonable density of each part of the course			
	Amount of exercise (0.26)	Reasonably-assigned amount of exercise for large,mediumand small exercise,and alternate it from small to large reasonably			
	Practice intensity (0.33)	Arrange the proper exercise intensity according to the content request,heart rate curve accords with science;the high point meets to the requirement			
Teaching goals (0.051)	Situation of marstering to class (0.68)	Students can marster the main content bassicly, and knoww the emphasis and difficult points clearly			
	Teaching purpose (0.32)	Finish the teaching purpose betterly; pay attention to individual development of students,master the basic technology and skills properly			
Total scores					
Advice					

Teacher in charge_____(Signature) Audit teacher_____(Signature)

Study on Improving the Soft Strength in Shaolin Wushu Gymnasium School

Bai Yun-qing

Huanghe Science and Technology College Zhengzhou Henan, China
byq@hhstu.edu.cn

Abstract. With the social progress, economic progress and gradual improvement of hardware facilities in Shaolin Wushu Gymnasium School, Soft strength will become its new developing direction. Combining the present developing situations of Shaolin Wushu Gymnasium School, and based on the specific conditions, the author puts forward that promoting the idea for running schools, managing them scientifically, stressing their characteristics and setting examples for others should be the central contents of improving the soft strength in Shaolin Wushu Gymnasium School.

Keywords: Shaolinsi Wushu Gymnasium School, Soft strength research.

1   Introduction

The term of "Soft Strength", which originally derived from a international terminology, was firstly introduced by Joseph·Nile, the minister of the Political College at Harvard University during the late 1980s of the 20th century. Soft Power, which is referred to as a kind of intangible spirit that can affect other nation's will, includes the attraction of political system, magnetism of worth, affection of culture, persuasion of diplomacy, international renown and the fascination of people's image. "Soft Strength" is stated as oppose to Hard Strength. If Hard Power is related to more visible power, Soft Strength shows more invisible feature. The idea of Soft Strength appeared early in ancient China, which is reflected mainly in the philosophy of Taoism. Taking the words from LaoZi for example, it says: "the softest thing in the world dashed against and overcomes the hardest". And "the soft wins over the hard". Both the wisdom of "respecting the soft" and the advocate of Soft Power mean the partiality for tender power.

In the 21st century, we have great economic boom. As a special training center for the talents, Shaolin Wushu Gymnasium School is playing irreplaceable role in our country and society. Especially after the reform and opening, the tide of practicing martial art has reached its peak after the movie The Shaolin Temple got its hot shot on screen. And it has become a general trend for the contemporary youth to learn Kongfu in Shaolin Temple. Numerous local schools sprang up like the mushroom, but driven by the economic benefit, some speculators who know nothing about the martial art also launched their course. It is dirty, messy and bad, which heavily damage the image of Shaolin Temple. In order to standardize the Wushu Gymnasium School's development and get rid of the potential risks, in 1985, the Shaolin Wushu Administration Office was

L. Qi (Ed.): PDCN 2010, CCIS 137, pp. 110–115, 2011.

established by Dengfeng Country Government with the involvement of Sports Committee, Education Council and Police office. It is aimed at making a general regulation of running the Wushu Gymnasium School within Dengfeng Area. Based on careful survey and investigation, in 1990 the government issued No.32 document of the Announcement about Strengthening the Administration of Wushu Gymnasium School, defined the inform pattern of the approving to the school building by Sports Council, and unified the rules of management and made "the Six Rules" for it. With those above, the school launching is becoming more and more standardized. Today the school's buildings attract an increasing attention from people for the sake of social development. And whether they can provide talents to the society nor not has become an important social problem, which has direct relation to their survival and prospective. Therefore, to cover the social need and push forward a steady Wushu industry, inner building should be the next focus of attention as well as its soft strength, and it has already become an important task for the contemporary Wushu education.

2   Promoting School Running Concept and Making School Spirit Are the Most Important Strategy to Promote the Soft Strength of the Martial Art School

School-running concept is a flag that shows its distinguished feature to the society and also is a program that integrates ideas and actions. It is not only a summary of the martial art development in the past, but also a future goal of its development. The advanced school-running concept is base on the deep recognition of the regular education pattern and the epoch characteristics. It is the essence of the whole educational system which precipitates the school's historical traditions, and reflects the school's social background and the common hope of the headmaster and the teacher. And the same time, it is also the reason, the motivation and the hope of the school' running. Once it is recognized or widely spread in the society, it will stand outside from lots of the same type schools and become a unique brand school. Then it will play a decisive role and give scope to its massive strength in the near- equal hardware competition. In order to promote the school-running concept, there are several aspects needed to do well: firstly, summarize the situation of the school's development, recall the school's running history, choose the useful experience, and review the problems existed during the process of developing, then find out the corresponding policies, promote its school-running concept of "to grow up--- to be talented--- to succeed"; secondly, analyze the current atmosphere of the Martial arts school, find out the advantages and disadvantages, opportunities and challenges of the other schools. And set the practical train of thought of development, development direction and value pursuit. Thirdly, the businessman of martial arts schools should study and discuss widely, develop the different level discussions, listen to different ideas of different people, negotiate with the experts and then get benefit advice, achieve the consensus according to the practical situation at last. Fourthly, reasonably state the school-running concept of "to grow up--- to be talented--- to succeed", making it inclusive be worth reading, and expressing various thoughts and values. "To grow up" means to let the student who study in the martial arts school learn how to be a real man under the principle of "education bring up people" giving them virtue education, law education, safety education and so on, especially to those "problem children." "To be talented" is base on "to grow up", giving different students different lessons to make them gain a special skill. "To succeed" means the martial arts school provides the student the student the opportunities of job-hunting so that they can find their real value after gaining the special skill. Fifthly, inspect the reasonableness of the school- running concept during the education practice according to the school reality, inspect whether the concept is right or not, whether it reflect the innate character and regular pattern of education, whether it accord with the basic character of the school, the make corresponding adjustment and try to realize the good interaction of the school-running practice and concept.

3   Insisting People-Oriented Principle and Scientific Management Is the Strong Point of Labor Power to Compact the Softer Power of the Martial Art School

The management patterns of the martial art school are mostly the type of clan in the past. with the continuing development and increasing demands from social needs, there is a gradual transition towards the common school on the management pattern of the martial art school. The martial art schools use the president's responsibility system, which means that the headmaster manage all teachings, all administration and logistics management and so on. Fewer martial art schools adopt the board of directors leading system, but it is not practical. The members of the board are mostly the clan members. Even if there are employees, they merely come up with their own advice without putting it into practice, since the chairman determines everything at last. That is the system of "president's responsibility system" in fact. Human resource is always the key, whatever the management pattern is or whoever manages the school. The goal of management is to give full play to human's value and potential. The human management is the blend of review and action, attention and advice, leading and construction, co-working and negotiation, stimulation and inspiration, believing and respect, interaction and dependence, leniency and democracy, mind and concept. Everyone has his or her own contribution, which brings the new epoch intension and harmonious developing motivation to the management pattern, thus forming the common value pursuit between different members. What's more, once combining this type of management pattern with human's value pursuit, the martial art school will get inexhaustible resource and wisdom.

It is necessary to do well in "Three Innate Quality" and "Five Insistence" to implement the new humanistic management. Firstly, promote the coaches and the teachers' virtue, their teaching ability, teaching attitude and the students' studying atmosphere, behavior and their great ideals; promote the staff's service attitude and their sense of responsibility and so on. This is a person's originally standing foundation, also is the basic strength of an organization. Secondly, try to reinforce the quality of unity, harmony, honesty and dedication. Thirdly, improve the headmasters' quality; mostly improve the leader's ability of making policy and management strategic. The headmasters are the decision-makers of guiding ideology and other aspects of daily management system; the headmasters' qualities influence the school's development directly. "Five Insistences" is the policy which means putting the student in the first place, doing what the student need and trying to provide all for students, to serve all student, and to insure student's all". Insist "talents strengthen school", establish "famous school with excellent teachers" and form the good atmosphere of training and studying. Nowadays, the students choose not only the famous schools, but also the excellent teachers, and the good teacher not only "obtain twice the result with half the effort", but also give the active influence on the student's growing-up. Insist on creating the career together; emphasize on making contributions in one's own position, practice in details, try to create the atmosphere of "competition in order, displaying one's talents fully". Insist on the positioning orientation, perfect the performance evaluation, specify the duty and responsibility, show one's strong points and hide one's weakness, plan to develop together; insist on the party construction, form excellent work style and harmonious developing atmosphere.

4 Strengthening the Brand Establishment and Highlighting the Distinctiveness Are the Two Brand-New Growing Points to Bring Up the Martial Art Schools' Soft Strength

The more mature a society is, the more remarkable its brand effect is. The education has come into the age of competition. "The great education" needs "the greater brand", "The greater brand" will promote a "greater development". It would be a paralysis for the publicly maintained martial art school, if they don't have an organized and meaningful plan for the brand, or they don't pay much attention to the brand consciousness and no efficient management. It can be also called a fatal point to them. Therefore, the brand is not only a profitable real worth but also an intangible asset to the martial art schools. It involves efforts in six aspects to establish the brand of martial art school. The first is accurate brand positioning. "Seeking for the exact position, highlighting the characteristics, and displaying the distinctiveness" is the basic three factors for the martial art school to be a brand school. The brand positioning should follow and consider fully the following principles, such as the objective demand of our society, the schools' basic foundation, the schools' objective conditions and the objective laws of education. Then we can find out our service objects and the exact brand position in the marketplace, thus building up our own key competitive abilities. The secondly is the stable cultivation pattern. The essence of a brand is actually a kind of promise, the process of practicing its promise. The foundation stone of a brand is its quality. The quality of students and the quality of training are the "brand" of martial art schools. The stable cultivation patterns, the sturdy teaching and practicing systems are the guarantees of a fulfilled quality promise of martial art schools. The third is the wide range of employment destination. The wide range of employment destination is the essence and soul of Martial art schools, it's not only deeply rooted in the school but also expand outside the schools. Basing on the actual situations of the students, order-mode education patterns is the essence of martial art schools, and the core strength of their victories. The Fourth is the long-term out matches. The existence of a martial art school brand is not decided by itself but the students and the parents. A successful brand also indicates a favorable social effect. The out match can not only build up images, but also provide a way to examine the training effect; moreover, it's also an efficient way to win the wide support of parents and the society. The fifth is the top-ranking faculties. The principal and teachers are the core and decisive factors to fulfill the cultivation objectives. The branded school cannot be separated from brand principal and brand teacher. "High quality of individual, well organized group and full of innovation spirits" are the demands for faculties, but also the important contents for martial art schools' brand. The sixth is Careful brand maintenance. It is difficult to create a brand and more difficult to maintain and promote a brand. Once a brand comes into being, the maintenance and development plan should be launched, while the key factors of maintenance is innovation. Once it lost, it would lose its advantage and become a non-brand in today's fierce competition.

5 Modeling the Public Image and Enlarging Its Popularity Are the Standpoints for Martial Art Schools' Settlement of Soft Strength

The pubic image is the reflection of social publics' attitude towards the external and internal characterizes of martial art schools, also is the public evaluation. The most important to build up a favorable image is to strengthen its "internal work", which is to improve the education quality, quality of personnel training and wide range of employment channels. At the same time, we should also bring in the concept and tactics of marketing promotion, which we can add them with our delicate scheme, elaborate package and careful operation, thus showing the world the favorable public image of martial art. However, some rules should be paid to the establishment of social image. We can publicize our school at high level starting point and all-round dimension from different and varied perspectives. Especially we should make full use of the modern science and technology to enhance the campus net construction in order to achieve the aim of building it into an information and resources center for the faculties' research and teaching, studying center for the students and also a clicking center for social communities. The second is to pay much attention to the establishment of teachers and students' image. Teachers and students are the spokesman of school's image; therefore much attention should be paid to the image establishment and behaviors guidance, which requires the teachers' image of dedicating themselves to their work, of taking delight from their work and of being professional towards their work. And the students are required to be united, progressive, cheerful in studying, responsible for the society, thus present themselves in the pubic, and build up the school's favorable image. Thirdly, much attention should be paid to the establishment of campus image. The campus image is a kind of sustainable education spirit and brand. Although the school's School principals, teachers, students often change, but the spirit keeps eternal, which always is the unexhausted motive force for the school's development. The school should actively lead their faculty to integrate the school's "working objective" and the educations' "ultimate value", and let the staff voluntarily participate in the establishment of the martial art schools' image on the premise of their understanding to the tasks and core value of education. Furthermore, we can intensify the acceptance of the society and parents towards the school' image, and foster the faculty to devote all their lifetime to the martial art career.

6 Conclusion

Above all, in the contemporary society, with high speed development of knowledge and economy, Shaolin Wushu Gymnasium Schools have stepped onto a new stage, and they are heading to the direction of diversification and industrialization. As an important institute of culture inheriting and talent training, the issue of soft strength building receives increasingly high attention. Nothing but having a further understanding to its connotation, recognizing the problems which exists in the developing process and finding out the accordingly efficient solution, we can better improve the development of the Shaolin Wushu Gymnasium School. To provide a strong intellectual support for the development of the social and Wushu development plays an important role in the arising of Wushu Schools.

References

1. Li, H.-s.: A Study on the Soft Strength of University. Fu Dan Education Forum 3(4) (2005) (in Chinese)
2. Wang, Z.-h., Cai, B.: Research on School Wushu and Its Activity Changes in Contemporary China. Journal of Beijing Sport University (April 2004) (in Chinese)
3. Ma, Y.-f., The Situation Problems and Measures on Wushu School. Sports Culture Guide, 14–16 (December 2005) (in Chinese)
4. Liu, H.-c.: Study on the Wushu Education History and Development. Sports & Science, 78–80 (May 2004) (in Chinese)
5. Li, Y., Zhao, Z.: Present situation of the Chinese Wushu schools and the countermeasures. Journal of WuHan Institute of Physical Education, 27–29 (June 2003) (in Chinese)
6. Liu, Y.: Research on The Current Situation and Development Strategy on the Running of Wushu Schools in Shandong Province. Journal of Beijing Sport University, 1406–1408 (October 2005) (in Chinese)
7. Guo, L., Li, J.: Investigation on Current Situation of Wushu Institutes in Shanxi Province, China Sport Science and Technology, 53–55 (November 2003) (in Chinese)

The Factors Influencing the Employment of National Traditional Sports (NTS) Gradutes in Henan Province and Countermeasures

Zemin Xiao

Henan Vocational and Technical College, Zhengzhou, Henan, China
hezhixiaozemin@126.com

Abstract. Based on the analysis of the factors influencing the employment of NTS graduates in Henan Province, the thesis gives corresponding suggestions and countermeasures upon the main problems existing in the training and employment of NTS professionals in Henan Province, and provides theoretical reference for the training mode and adjustment of curriculum setting for NTS professionals in Henan Province.

Keywords: strength, the load combination method, horizontally vertically.

1 Introduction

In 1998, the major of martial arts is adjusted to "NTS" by the Ministry of Education, including three orientations, i.e. martial arts, traditional sports health preservation, and national folk sports, which not only broadened the professional size of the former major of martial arts, but also rose the position and role of NTS in the physical education in China's universities. At present, there are five universities in Henan Province which set the major of NTS, namely, Henan University, Henan Normal University, Physical Education College of Zhengzhou University, Luoyang Normal University, and Huanghe University of Technology. With the expansion of enrollment, there will be a large number of professionals of the major serving the society. To a certain extent, the quality of the professionals and the employment situation of the graduates greatly determine the development direction and vitality of the major, therefore, in order to maintain the sustainable development of the major and meet the actual demand of the society, it is necessary to research the employment trends and status of the students majoring in national traditional sports.

2 Research Object and Methods

2.1 The Graduates and Partial Students in School of the Five Universities with the Major of NTS

2.2 Research Methods

Documents, interviews with experts, logical analysis etc.

L. Qi (Ed.): PDCN 2010, CCIS 137, pp. 116–120, 2011.

3 Research Results and Analysis

3.1 Employment Characteristics of NTS in Henan Province

3.1.1 Severe Employment Situation

Since the Ministry of Education defined the plan of expanding university students' enrollment in 1998, the graduates have increased sharply. In addition to the external factors including enterprise restructuring, the increasing of off-work persons, the transfer of rural surplus labor force and others, the employment situation for current university graduates is hard. The sharp increase of conflicts within a short time is bound to affect the social harmony and healthy development of higher education, and relate to the country's stability and happiness of the families. How to do well the work upon the employment of the university students under the new situation has become the important issues of the universities and relevant departments.

The employment situation of the graduates from the physical education departments of Henan Province is severer. As enrollment continues to expand, this situation is bound to worsen the employment situation of physical education graduates in Henan Province. The digestion ability of employment market of physical education in Henan Province is limited. Except physical education teachers and related sports industry, the graduates are few employed in other fields, so, the NTS graduates are facing serious employment pressure.

3.1.2 Characteristics of Regional Differences in Employment

In course of analyzing and forecasting objective environment, it is found that the environment and actual conditions has regional characteristics and differences. I have deeply felt the differences in growing experience, characters, ideology, family concepts, employment concepts and psychology in the practical student management work. After talking and visiting, I find that the people in Henan Province are comparatively conservative in the employment of the major of NTS. Most parents hope their children to work nearby, unwilling to work far away from home, which will definitely affect the flexibility of employment of the graduates.

A survey shows that over 90% of the NTS graduates hope to work in the big or medium sized cities, while few are willing to work in other provinces or remote areas, from which we can find that the traditional concepts of human and geography have affected the employment rate of NTS graduates.

3.1.3 Narrow Careers Choosing

NTS is closely linked with social needs and its training objective and curriculum settings must be consistent with the needs and development of the society. However, NTS does not have its unique professional features. Its curriculum and content settings are mainly martial arts, which have limited the diversity of the students' system of knowledge. The single professional knowledge of sports is bound to affect the broadness of employment. The employment channel is relatively narrow, and the employment has the characteristics of singleness.

According to investigation, it is found that 80% of the NTS graduates are willing to engage in fitness coaching, sports teaching, etc. Under current severe situation of employment, if the students can not shake off the shackles of their own major, it will be hard for them to be employed. Of course, such long-standing condition relates with the employment guidance of the school and curriculum teaching on career planning and the students' closed concepts of employment choosing. Especially in recent years, with the continued enrollment expansion of the universities and the upgrading of junior college education into undergraduate education, under the premise of increasing enrollment while comparatively decreasing of employers, the employment of the graduates have met unprecedented difficulties.

3.1.4 Characteristics of High Employment Expectations

Every one dreams and expects a good career in the future. The university is the connection stage between school and society, and a person will realize the role transition from a student to a social person. The investigation shows that, 70% of the students want to work in public institutions, and the most desirable job is physical education teacher; the second one is to do business, accounting for 10%. With the development of market economy, the difficulty of employment is increasing, and more and more students gradually established their own businesses, which is related to the supporting of the state in policy and the good quality of the physical education students including teamwork, agility, active and self-confidence; 12% want to work as a public servant; for the rest 8%, some want to develop in physical bodybuilding clubs and other physical education industries; in addition, it is found from the investigation of employment choosing motives that most graduates take welfare and treatment, career development and social position as the first motive. The high expectation of pursing blindly high income and position while ignoring self strong points and pursuing blindly personal interest while neglecting the conflicts between the interests and social reality are disadvantageous to employment.

3.1.5 Diversified Forms of Employment

With the continuing perfection of social market economy system, viewing from the relationship between professionals and careers, they have both linkages and differences. The survey and visiting shows that many NTS graduates have engaged in wider careers, such as advertising design, marketing, services, army and so on. Nowadays, it is very common for cross-professional employment, but what learnt in the university is not used in the work, which is new topic for the education and teaching reform of the universities. In addition, under the condition that the state has issued many policies good for the employment of university graduates, the employment of the graduates has the characteristics of diversified forms. The employment ways of NTS graduates are more flexible and diversified, such as working as a teacher in rural areas, taking national public servant enrollment examination, self business establishment, taking postgraduate entrance examination, etc. Of course, the diversity of employment scope and forms is the inevitable trend for the employment of NTS graduates, which is good to the society, university, family and personal development to a certain extent.

3.1.6 Lack of Comprehensive Ability of Practice

The talk, consultancy, investigation and research to the experts and employers of NTS show that the comprehensive ability of practice of NTS graduates are not ideal. The employers think that the students are good in professional skills, common in the ability of teaching, training and organization, and bad in scientific research, innovation and self restriction. It is mainly because that most students are from martial arts schools or sports school, and the results of cultural courses are comparatively low. While after they enter the university, most of them still have not transferred their concepts to adapt to the university's education mode of comprehensive quality training. They still think that they shall mainly pay attention to technical training, therefore the emphasis on study and improvement of theoretical accomplishment is inadequate, which is especially serious in freshman and sophomore years. So, in order to adapt to the social development in the 21st century and the requirement of high quality talents, firstly, the NTS students shall change completely their concepts, pay more attention to the learning of basic theory, the overall training and improvement of comprehensive quality in all-round way, and secondly, make a good position for the object and clarify the direction of efforts, and constantly improve the overall ability of practice and innovative ability.

4 Countermeasures of Improving Employment Rate of NTS Students

4.1 Restrict School Size and Reduce Employment Pressure

The education sectors of Henan Province should strengthen review power based on the demand of the society to NTS talents, and evaluate the qualification of the universities in setting the major of NTS, adopting the mechanism of the survival of the fittest. For those not qualified for running or having serious problems in the running, the qualification of running should be cancelled; these powerful measures can restrict running scale, release the conflicts between the supply and demand, and relieve the employment pressure of NTS graduates.

4.2 Explore Employment Space and Broaden Employment Channels

With the continuing development and progress of China's economy, the cause of physical education is showing a thriving scene. Martial arts industry and service industries develop rapidly, resulting in a number of related jobs which can be chosen by the graduates. Therefore, NTS students should strive to expand their own knowledge, improve their own ability and make themselves compound talents of "one professional and multi-skills", clarify future employment direction under the premise of adapting to social demand and seeking more joints between the major and post, which can both solve the problem of employment and realize professional ideal.

4.3 Change Employment Concepts and Go to the West

The graduates should judge rightly their own severe situation of employment, change their own concept of employment choosing, while can not aim too high and blindly follow. They should evaluate their own conditions rationally and objectively, position the employment scientifically, and adjust at the right time according to the actual conditions and rationally reduce the expectation to the employment. Go to the west and grassroots units, maybe they can fully exert their own strong points and realize their own ideals there.

4.4 Strengthen Information Communication and Employment Guidance

The universities should strengthen their connection with all the circles of the society, strive to explore employment market, adopt the method of "go out of the campus and invite the employers to come in" to strengthen the contact and communication with the employers, know timely the employment information of relevant units, and recommend graduates to the employers for practice or interview so as to create more chances of employment for the graduates.

4.5 Form Its Own Characteristics of Running and Improve the Comprehensive Quality of the Students

For the major of NTS, the universities must adapt to market demand, adjust development ideas of the major, speed up major settings and the adjustment of professional structure with priority, integrate teaching resources, increase the courses adapting to the demand of social development and closely relating to employment, realize the talents training mechanism of multi-discipline and cross-major for physical education and meet the demand of the students of different levels and demands. The universities should also improve teaching quality, reform teaching contents, method and measure, exert its own advantages, strengthen the training mode with the characteristics of the university, improve the comprehensive quality of the students to make the students master both sufficient professional basic knowledge and skills and be skilled in relevant knowledge and skills, thus making the students transfer into the compound talents with the characteristics of "thick foundation, wide caliber, strong ability, high innovation and wide adaptation", which is advantageous for improving the competitiveness of job choosing and employment and expand employment channels.

References

1. 2006 Annual Report upon University Graduate's Employment Situation and Development [OL] (2006),
   http://www.biz.163.com/06/0403/18/2DQAN7R500020QDS.html
2. An Employment Survey upon the Post of Physical Education Teacher Eager for More Undergraduate Graduates [N / OL]. China Sports Newspaper,
   http://www.sports.cn/
3. State Council: Seven Measures to Promote the Employment of University Graduates [OL],
   http://www.edu.cn/zong_he_news_465/20090108/t20090108_353104.shtml

Author Index

GPSR Compliance

*The European Union's (EU) General Product Safety Regulation (GPSR)
is a set of rules that requires consumer products to be safe and our
obligations to ensure this.*

*If you have any concerns about our products, you can contact us on
ProductSafety@springernature.com*

In case Publisher is established outside the EU, the EU authorized
representative is:

Springer Nature Customer Service Center GmbH
Europaplatz 3
69115 Heidelberg, Germany

Batch number: 09478804

Printed by Printforce, the Netherlands